PETERSON'S®

MASTER THE™ CNA & HHA EXAMS®

1ST EDITION

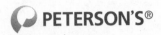 **PETERSON'S®**

About Peterson's®

Peterson's has been your trusted educational publisher for more than 50 years. It's a milestone we're quite proud of as we continue to offer the most accurate, dependable, high-quality educational content in the field, providing you with everything you need to succeed. No matter where you are on your academic or professional path, you can rely on Peterson's for its books, online information, expert test-prep tools, the most up-to-date education exploration data, and the highest quality career success resources—everything you need to achieve your education goals. For our complete line of products, visit **www.petersons.com.**

For more information or to give us feedback, contact Peterson's, 4380 S. Syracuse Dr., Denver, CO 80237; 800-338-3282 Ext. 54229; or visit us online at **www.petersons.com.**

NCSBN® is a registered trademark of the National Council of State Boards of Nursing, Inc. (NCSBN®), which did not collaborate in the development of, and does not endorse, this product.

ISBN-13: 978-0-7689-4576-8

Printed in the United States of America

10 9 8 7 6 5 4 3 2 1   23 22 21

First Edition

CONTENTS

PART I: THE CERTIFIED NURSING ASSISTANT AND HOME HEALTH AIDE PROFESSIONS AND THEIR EXAMS

01 | INTRODUCTION TO THE CNA AND HHA PROFESSIONS   2

CONTENTS

CONTENTS

BEFORE YOU BEGIN

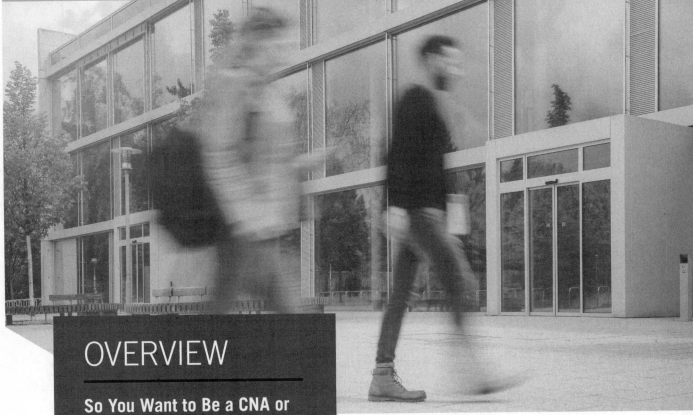

OVERVIEW

SO YOU WANT TO BE A CNA OR HHA

If you are looking for a career where you have the opportunity to truly make a difference in the lives of patients and clients, studying to become a certified nursing assistant or aide (CNA) or a home health assistant or aide (HHA) is an excellent choice. The educational path to becoming a CNA or HHA is typically affordable and can be completed in a relatively short amount of time. Because patient care is usually needed around the clock, CNAs and HHAs often work in a wide variety of positions and locations and can work day, night, and weekend shifts.

According to the U.S. Bureau of Labor Statistics (BLS), it is a great time to be a CNA or an HHA!

The BLS projected that there would be approximately 174,000 job openings for CNAs/HHAs **each year** between 2019 and 2029. With advances in medicine and patient care, the population of older citizens in our country increases every year. When you combine a large aging population with a nationwide shortage of nurses across all levels of nursing, it creates a high level of job security in these positions now through the end of the decade.

Peterson's *Master the™ CNA & HHA Exams®* is written for candidates hoping to pass the CNA or HHA examinations. This book gives you the most thorough review and test-like practice available, covering all the categories and subcategories tested on the exam.

Who Should Use This Book?

Peterson's *Master the™ CNA & HHA Exams®* is a valuable resource in your certification journey if you can answer "yes" to the following statements:

- You want to prepare for your certification exam in your own time and at your own pace, but you don't have time for a test preparation program that takes weeks to complete.

- You want a guide that covers all the key points you need to know but doesn't waste time on topics you don't absolutely have to know for the exam.

- You want a collection of practice CNA/HHA exams that look like the tests you will actually take to increase your chances of passing the exam.

How This Book Is Organized

Peterson's *Master the™ CNA & HHA Exams®* is divided into four parts to help you understand the role of the certified nursing assistant, the structure of the CNA and HHA examinations, and what you need to know to pass them and obtain licensure. Full-length practice tests are included to help test your knowledge and provide a basis for creating a study plan.

Part I (Chapter 1) gives you a quick overview of the important facts you need to know about the CNA and HHA professions, the current structure of certification exams, CNA/HHA job descriptions, and the current outlook for these careers.

Part II (Chapter 2) contains a brief pre-test designed to help you identify those areas where you need to spend more time in your review sessions.

Part III (Chapters 3–8) reviews the following Client Needs categories and subcategories found on the current CNA Test Plan:

> Chapter 3—Foundations: Anatomy, Physiology, and Medical Terminology
>
> Chapter 4—Roles of the CNA and HHA
>
> Chapter 5—Activities of Daily Living
>
> Chapter 6—Basic Nursing Skills
>
> Chapter 7—Psychosocial Care Skills

Part IV includes three full-length practice tests that simulate the exam topics and structure, so you're fully prepared for test day.

Part V (Helpful Information for Prospective CNAs and HHAs) provides supplemental information on state boards of nursing and professional organizations as well as websites you can check for health, education, and job information.

How to Use This Book

Review Part I to familiarize yourself with the CNA and HHA professions and career outlooks. Part I will also provide you with the opportunity to review the CNA Test Plan. Proven test-taking strategies and study techniques are provided along with our top 10 strategies for choosing the correct answer.

Take the Pre-Test in Part II. This brief test is designed to replicate the types of questions you will find on the actual CNA exam, only in a shortened format. We've provided detailed answer explanations for all answer choices so that you can review why an answer was correct or incorrect. Use these as a starting point to tailor your study plan.

Review the chapters in Part III. Each chapter covers one of the Client Needs categories and its subcategories, reviewing the major concepts you will need to know to pass the CNA exam. Before you dive into a chapter, skim the bulleted overview, which lists the topics covered in the chapter. At the end of every review section or chapter, you will find practice questions along with detailed answer explanations. Use these questions to test your understanding and further assess where you will need to focus your study plan. The Summing It Up sections at the end of each chapter provide a "highlight reel" of the concepts discussed in that chapter.

Take the practice tests in Part IV under test-like conditions. As you finish each practice test, check your answers against the answer keys and read the explanation for each question you missed. If you have the time, read all the answer explanations—they're great for a more in-depth CNA review. You can use your results from these practice tests to identify your strengths and weaknesses, and then spend the rest of your time leading up to your exam reviewing the areas where you need the most improvement.

Reference the supplemental material in Part V as needed for more information on professional organizations and helpful websites to enhance your learning experience and expand your knowledge base.

Proven Strategies to Raise Your Score

In taking the CNA & HHA exams, some strategies are more useful than others. The following tips will help you pass the exam.

1 **Create a study plan and stick to it.** The right study plan will help you get the most out of this book in the time that you have.

2 **Review key test elements daily for several weeks before the exam.** Reread the Test Plan to be sure that you understand the categories and subcategories on the exams.

3 **Complete all the exercises in this book.** Doing so will help you recognize your areas of strength and discover which areas need improvement.

4 **If possible, visit the test center before the day of the exam.** This will help you become familiar with the location and how long it takes to travel there. On the day of the exam, leave plenty of time to get to the test center in case the buses/subways/ trains are running late, the weather is bad, or parking your car is a problem.

5 **Avoid cramming the night before the exam.** This will only make you feel more nervous. It is not likely to help you learn enough to make a difference on your test score.

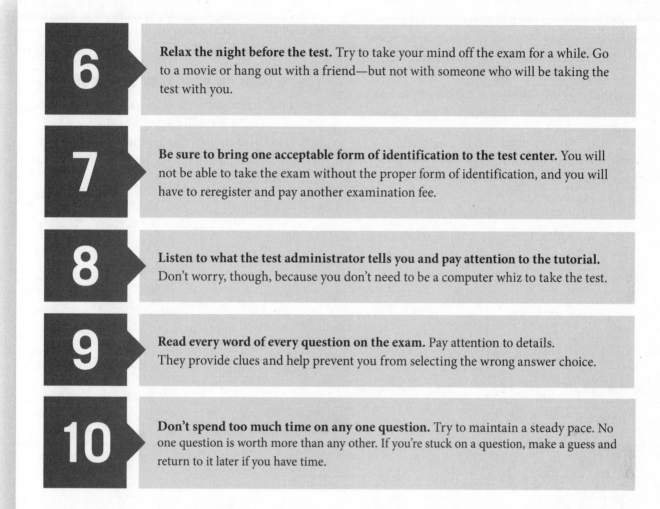

6   **Relax the night before the test.** Try to take your mind off the exam for a while. Go to a movie or hang out with a friend—but not with someone who will be taking the test with you.

7   **Be sure to bring one acceptable form of identification to the test center.** You will not be able to take the exam without the proper form of identification, and you will have to reregister and pay another examination fee.

8   **Listen to what the test administrator tells you and pay attention to the tutorial.** Don't worry, though, because you don't need to be a computer whiz to take the test.

9   **Read every word of every question on the exam.** Pay attention to details. They provide clues and help prevent you from selecting the wrong answer choice.

10   **Don't spend too much time on any one question.** Try to maintain a steady pace. No one question is worth more than any other. If you're stuck on a question, make a guess and return to it later if you have time.

Print or Online? You Decide!

Take your test-prep experience online and on the go for automated-timing, instant feedback, and scoring results. Go to Petersons.com and subscribe to gain instant access to digital versions of the tests in this book, 3 additional CNA/HHA practice tests, and much more.

Special Study Features

Master the™ CNA & HHA Exams® is designed to be as user-friendly as it is complete. To this end, it includes several features to make your preparation more efficient.

Overview

Each chapter begins with a bulleted overview listing the topics that are covered in the chapter. This will help you find content for the major aspects of the certification exams and also allow you to quickly find content to brush up on any content "weak areas" you might have.

Summing It Up

Each review chapter ends with a point-by-point summary that captures the most important information in the chapter. The summaries are a convenient way to review the main points one last time before the exam.

Give Us Your Feedback

Peterson's publishes a full line of books—test prep, education exploration, financial aid, and career preparation. Peterson's publications can be found at high school guidance offices, college libraries and career centers, and your local bookstore and library. In addition, you can find Peterson's products online at **www. petersons.com**.

We welcome any comments or suggestions you may have about this publication. Please call our customer service department at 800-338-3282 Ext. 54229 or send an email message to custsvc@petersons.com. Your feedback will help us make educational dreams possible for you—and others like you.

You're Well on Your Way to Success!

Remember that knowledge is power. Using *Master the™ CNA & HHA Exams*® will help you become familiar with the kind of content that appears in actual exams. We look forward to helping you obtain your certification. Good luck!

PART I

THE CERTIFIED NURSING ASSISTANT AND HOME HEALTH AIDE PROFESSIONS AND THEIR EXAMS

1 | Introduction to the CNA and HHA Professions

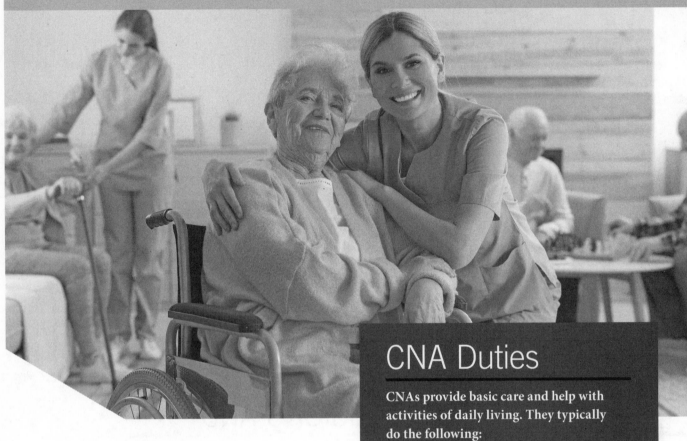

CNA Duties

CNAs provide basic care and help with activities of daily living. They typically do the following:

- Clean and bathe patients
- Help patients use the toilet and dress
- Turn, reposition, and transfer patients between beds and wheelchairs
- Listen to and record patients' health concerns and report that information to nurses
- Measure patients' vital signs, such as blood pressure and temperature
- Serve meals and help patients eat
- Help patients to move around the facility, such as by pushing their wheelchairs
- Clean equipment and facilities
- Change linens
- Stock supplies

CNA OR HHA? AND WHAT'S THE DIFFERENCE?

CNA and HHA job duties can be similar in many ways. Both offer basic care to their patients or clients, including changing bedding, assisting with bathing, dressing, grooming, and other routine tasks. While an HHA provides help with things like laundry, grocery-shopping, and taking patients for a walk, CNA job duties include slightly more advanced medical care. A CNA will monitor oxygen levels and vital signs, administer medications prescribed by a physician, dress sutures and change wound bandages—under the direction of a registered nurse or doctor. Furthermore, some of the typical duties of a CNA/HHA will vary further depending on where you're located, so it is important that you research and become familiar with your state's educational and certification requirements for both CNA and HHA.

WHAT NURSING ASSISTANTS OR CERTIFIED NURSING AIDES (CNAs) DO

CNAs, or nursing assistants or nurse aides, help patients with activities of daily living like eating and bathing. They provide basic care and help transport patients and clean treatment areas. Depending on their training level and the state in which they work, nursing assistants also may dispense medication. CNAs are often the principal caregivers in nursing and residential care facilities and can develop helpful relationships with their patients because some patients stay in these facilities for months or years.

Injuries and Illnesses

CNAs and HHAs have one of the highest rates of injuries and illnesses of all occupations. These workers frequently move patients and have other physically demanding tasks. They typically get training in how to properly lift people, which can reduce the risk of injury to both the patient and the caretaker. Adequate control of infection is an equally-important element of patient and staff safety, so hand-washing and other protocols to stop the spread of germs are key. In addition, CNAs/HHAs may work with clients who display difficult or violent behavior due to mental health or cognitive impairments. Aides also face hazards from minor infections and exposure to a number of diseases but can lessen their chance of infection by following proper hand-washing and other infection-control procedures.

Work Schedules

Although most CNAs and HHAs work full time, some work part time. Because nursing and residential care facilities and hospitals provide care at all hours, nursing assistants and HHAs may need to work nights, weekends, and holidays.

HOW TO BECOME A CNA

After graduating high school, aspiring CNAs typically must complete a state-approved education program and pass their state's competency exam. HHAs typically have at least a high school diploma or equivalent.

Education and Training

CNAs often need to complete a state-approved education program that includes both instruction on the principles of nursing and supervised clinical work. These programs are available in high schools, community colleges, vocational and technical schools, hospitals, and nursing homes.

In addition, nursing assistants typically complete a brief period of on-the-job training to learn about their specific employer's policies and procedures.

Important Qualities of a CNA

COMMUNICATION SKILLS Nursing assistants must listen and respond to patients' concerns. They also need to share information with other healthcare workers.	**PHYSICAL STAMINA** Nursing assistants spend much of their time on their feet. They must be able to perform tasks such as lifting or moving patients.
PATIENCE The routine tasks of cleaning, feeding, and bathing patients may be stressful. Nursing assistants must be able to complete these tasks with professionalism.	**COMPASSION** Nursing assistants help and care for people who are sick, injured, or need aid for other reasons. They need an empathetic attitude to do their work.

Licenses, Certifications, and Registrations

Specific requirements for nursing assistants vary by state. Nursing assistants often need a state-issued license or certification. After completing an approved education program, nursing assistants often must pass a competency exam, which allows them to use state-specific titles. Nursing assistants who have passed the competency exam are placed on a state registry. They must be on the state registry to work in a nursing home. Some states have other requirements as well, such as continuing education and a criminal background check. Check with state boards of nursing or health for more information. In some states, nursing assistants may earn additional credentials, such as Certified Medication Assistant (CMA). As a CMA, they may dispense medications.

WORK OUTLOOK

Nursing assistants held about 1.5 million jobs in 2019. The largest employers of nursing assistants were as follows:

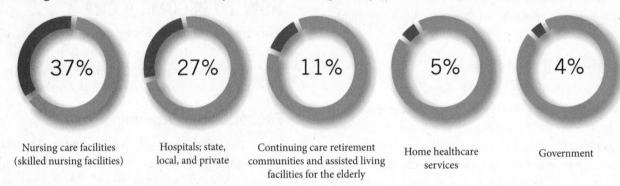

37%	27%	11%	5%	4%
Nursing care facilities (skilled nursing facilities)	Hospitals; state, local, and private	Continuing care retirement communities and assisted living facilities for the elderly	Home healthcare services	Government

The median annual wage for nursing assistants was $30,850 in May 2020. The median wage is the wage at which half the workers in an occupation earned more than that amount and half earned less. The lowest 10% earned less than $22,750, and the highest 10% earned more than $42,110.

In May 2020, the median annual wages for CNAs in the top industries in which they worked were as follows:

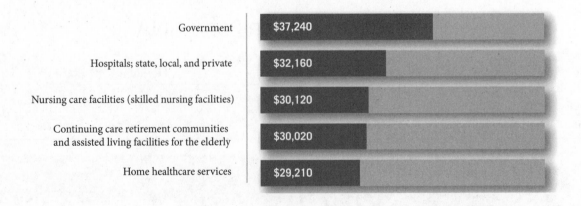

Government	$37,240
Hospitals; state, local, and private	$32,160
Nursing care facilities (skilled nursing facilities)	$30,120
Continuing care retirement communities and assisted living facilities for the elderly	$30,020
Home healthcare services	$29,210

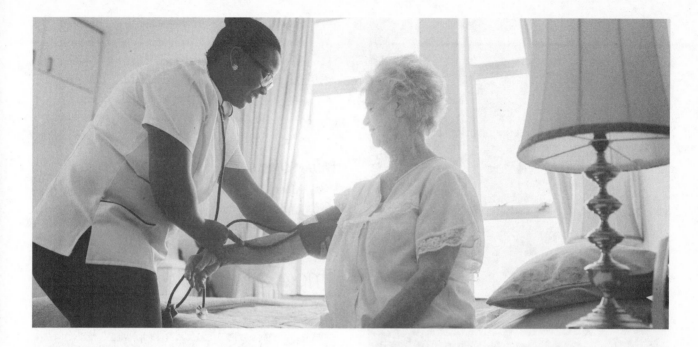

WHAT HOME HEALTH AIDES (HHAs) DO

Home health aides, assist clients in everyday tasks. Home health aides monitor the condition of people with disabilities or chronic illnesses and help them with daily living activities. They often help older adults who need assistance. Under the direction of a nurse or other healthcare practitioner, home health aides may be allowed to give a client medication or to check the client's vital signs.

HHAs may provide some basic health-related services—such as checking a client's pulse, temperature, and respiration rate—depending on the state in which they work. They also may help with simple prescribed exercises and with giving medications. Occasionally, they change bandages or dressings, give massages, care for skin, or help with braces and artificial limbs. With special training, experienced HHAs also may help with medical equipment, such as ventilators to help clients breathe.

HHAs are supervised by medical practitioners, usually nurses, and may work with therapists and other medical staff. These aides keep records on the client, such as services received, condition, and progress. They report changes in the client's condition to a supervisor or case manager.

HHA Duties

Home health aides typically do the following:

- **Assist clients in their daily personal tasks, such as bathing or dressing**
- **Perform housekeeping tasks, such as laundry, washing dishes, and vacuuming**
- **Help to organize a client's schedule and plan appointments**
- **Arrange transportation to doctors' offices or other outings**
- **Shop for groceries and prepare meals to meet a client's dietary specifications**
- **Keep clients engaged in their social networks and communities**

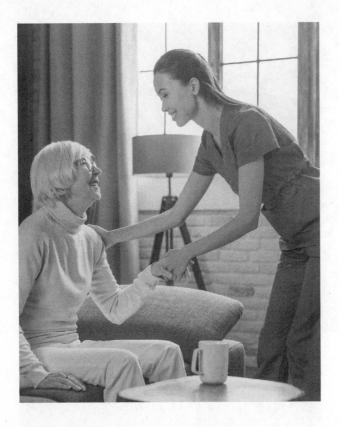

Work Environment

Many aides work in clients' homes; others work in group homes or care communities. Home health aides held about 3.4 million jobs in 2019.

- Some aides work with only one client, while others work with groups of clients. They sometimes stay with one client on a long-term basis or for a specific purpose, such as hospice care. They may work with other aides in shifts so that the client always has an aide.
- Aides may travel as they help people with disabilities go to work and stay engaged in their communities.

Injuries and Illnesses

- Work as a home health or personal care aide can be physically and emotionally demanding. Because they often move clients into and out of bed or help with standing or walking, aides must use proper lifting techniques to guard against back injury.

- In addition, aides may work with clients who have cognitive impairments or mental health issues and who may display difficult or violent behaviors. Aides also face hazards from minor infections and exposure to communicable diseases but can lessen their chance of infection by following proper procedures.

Work Schedules

- Most aides work full time, although part-time work is common. They may work evening and weekend hours, depending on their clients' needs. Work schedules may vary.

Important Qualities of an HHA

DETAIL ORIENTED Home health aides must adhere to specific rules and protocols to help care for clients. They must carefully follow instructions that they receive from other healthcare workers, such as how to care for wounds.

EMOTIONAL SKILLS Home health aides must be sensitive to clients' needs, especially while in extreme pain or distress. Aides must be compassionate and enjoy helping people.

INTEGRITY Home health aides must be dependable and trustworthy so that clients and their families can rely on them. They also should be respectful when tending to personal activities, such as helping clients bathe.

INTERPERSONAL SKILLS Home health aides must be able to communicate with clients and other healthcare workers. They need to listen closely to what they are being told and convey information clearly.

PHYSICAL STAMINA Home health aides should be comfortable doing physical tasks. They might need to be on their feet for many hours or do strenuous tasks, such as lifting or turning clients.

HOW TO BECOME A HOME HEALTH AIDE

Depending on their state, home health aides require a combination of basic education, training, and licensing for employment.

Education

- Home health aides typically need a high school diploma or equivalent, but some positions do not require it. Those working in certified home health or hospice agencies must complete formal training and pass a standardized test.

Training

- Home health aides may be trained in housekeeping tasks, such as cooking for clients who have special dietary needs. Aides may learn basic safety techniques, including how to respond in an emergency. If state certification is required, specific training may be needed.

- Training may be completed on the job or through programs. Training typically includes learning about personal hygiene, reading and recording vital signs, infection control, and basic nutrition.

- In addition, individual clients may have preferences that aides need time to learn.

Licenses, Certifications, and Registrations

- Home health aides may need to meet requirements specific to the state in which they work. For example, some states require HHAs to have a license or certification, which may involve completing training and passing a background check and a competency exam. For more information, check with your state board of health.

- Certified home health or hospice agencies that receive payments from federally funded programs, such as Medicare, must comply with regulations regarding aides' employment. Private care agencies that do not receive federal funds may have other employment requirements that vary by state.

- Aides also may be required to obtain certification in first aid and cardiopulmonary resuscitation (CPR).

PAY

The median annual wage for home health aides was $27,080 in May 2020. The median wage is the wage at which half the workers in an occupation earned more than that amount and half earned less. The lowest 10% earned less than $20,130, and the highest 10% earned more than $36,990.

In May 2020, the median annual wages for home health aides in the top industries in which they worked were as follows:

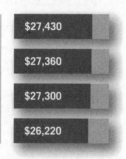

Continuing care retirement communities and assisted living facilities for the elderly	$27,430
Individual and family services	$27,360
Residential intellectual and developmental disability facilities	$27,300
Home healthcare services	$26,220

Most aides work full-time, although part-time work is common. They may work evening and weekend hours, depending on their clients' needs. Work schedules may vary.

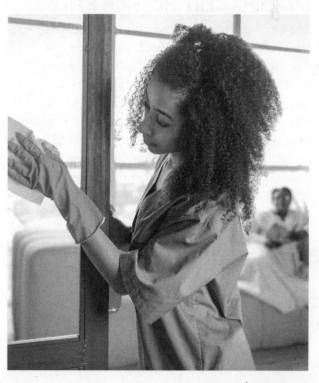

HOME HEALTH AIDES (HHAs) OCCUPATIONAL OUTLOOK

QUICK FACTS	
2020 Median Pay	$27,080 per year $13.02 per hour
Typical Entry-Level Education	High school diploma or equivalent
Work Experience in a Related Occupation	None
On-the-job Training	Short-term on-the-job training
Number of Jobs, 2019	3,439,700
Job Outlook, 2019-29	34% (Much faster than average)
Employment Change, 2019-29	Increase of 1,159,500 jobs

For additional information, see the *Bureau of Labor Statistics, U.S. Department of Labor, Occupational Outlook Handbook, Home Health and Personal Care Aides,* at **https://www.bls.gov/ooh/ healthcare/home-health-aides-and-personal-care-aides.htm.**

CNA/HHA CERTIFICATION EXAMS

The Certified Nursing Assistant (CNA) and Home Health Aide (HHA) exams are both multiple-choice standardized tests required by all 50 states to certify and license students that have completed the necessary training as designated by their state. There are two components to the most widely adopted licensing exams—the written test and the practical or skills test. The CNA and HHA certification exams have a lot of overlap, but there are a few minor differences. This section will cover the following areas:

- Training Requirements
- Written Test Overview and Topics
- Scoring
- The Practical Skills Exam
- Testing Logistics

TRAINING REQUIREMENTS

Both CNA and HHA candidates must attend and pass an approved training program that meets both the federal and state guidelines for their focus before they are eligible to sit for their licensing exam. There are national guidelines for both programs that require CNA/HHAs to complete a MINIMUM of 75 hours of training coupled with 16 hours of clinical experience in the field. However, many states (32 for CNA and 18 for HHA) have requirements that exceed this minimum, ranging from 76 to 180 hours of training and up to 100 hours of clinical experience. A quick online search will help you identify the most updated CNA/HHA requirements for your particular state. It is also important to make sure the CNA program you enroll in is approved by your state.

Other requirements include:

- Proof you're age 18 or older (some states allow 16 or 17-year-old applicants with parental consent)
- High school diploma or GED
- Valid driver's license or state ID
- CPR and first aid certification
- Physical exam
- Immunizations (vary by state regulations)
- Tuberculous test results
- Background check and fingerprinting

Not all HHA programs are regulated in the same way nationwide. Verify that your HHA training program is approved by your state by checking with your department of health.

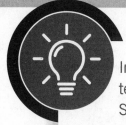

In some states, the written test can be administered in Spanish and/or orally if needed.

Written Test Overview and Topics

The CNA and HHA exams have many similarities, including exam topics and the length of the test. Although tests can vary by state, both tests are 60-70 questions with a 90-minute time limit. In addition, both tests require a practical skills exam that will be discussed in depth later in this section.

Both CNA and HHA licensing exams have similar topics related to patient care, ethics, legal issues, and roles and responsibilities. The CNA exam goes deeper and asks more technical questions; however, both exams focus on the same core topics.

EXAM TOPICS	
Activities of Daily Living	Resident Rights, Ethics and Legal Issues
Aging Process	Nutrition
Body Mechanics and Range of Motion	Roles and Responsibilities of the CNA/HHA
Communication	Safety
Cultural and Spiritual Needs	Infection Control
Mental Health	Vital Signs and Data Collection
Anatomy, Physiology, and Medical Terminology	

Core Topic Summaries

The most widely tested topics will be discussed at length throughout this book. The following are brief summaries of each topic:

1 **Activities of Daily Living (ADLs)**—This is the core function of the CNA/HHA position. ADLs include all the basic cares provided throughout the day including bathing, dressing, grooming, toileting, ambulating, and feeding.

2 **Aging Process**—This topic focuses on the aging process and how it affects body systems and the five senses.

3 **Anatomy, Physiology, and Medical Terminology**—This topic is an overview of the body, the systems within it, how they function to keep the body running, and common medical terminology connected with both of these positions.

4 **Body Mechanics and Range of Motion**—This topic includes body mechanics for proper lifting, transfers, etc., discussion about various tools and equipment used for these maneuvers, and range of motion vocabulary and best practices.

5 **Communication**—This topic discusses interpersonal communication with an emphasis on nonverbal communication as the main driver of how a person feels during communication interactions. Best practices for communicating with a variety of impaired patients are also included.

6 **Cultural and Spiritual Needs**—This topic covers various cultures, religions, and spiritual practices that CNAs/HHAs may encounter and how to be respectful while providing necessary care.

7 **Infection Control**—This topic is extremely important and includes an overview of the chain of infection, types of infections, handwashing, and best practices in the workplace.

8 **Mental Health**—This section discusses the most often occurring mental health issues, such as depression, anxiety, and mood disorders, and also memory-related disorders, such as dementia and Alzheimer's disease.

9 **Nutrition**—This topic covers an overview of nutrition and the national guidelines. It also includes a section about diet types (including mechanical soft, puree, etc.) and best practices on encouraging healthy diet choices for patients regardless of ability and understanding.

10 **Resident Rights, Ethics, and Legal Issues**—This topic focuses on resident and patient rights, ethics, and legal issues, including abuse, neglect, and abandonment. The topics of Long-Term Care Ombudsman, Adult Protective Services, and licensing requirements are also covered.

11 **Roles and Responsibilities of the CNA/HHA**—This section focuses on the scope of practice relating to the CNA/HHA and how to handle situations that go beyond your role.

12 **Safety Measures**—This section covers basic emergency preparedness, CPR and First Aid, and Personal Protective Equipment (PPE).

13 **Vital Signs and Data Collection**—This topic reviews important vital signs you should understand, including blood pressure, respiration, and oxygen saturation and discusses necessary data collection protocols for both CNAs and HHAs.

SCORING

Scoring for both the CNA and HHA exams is based on a traditional percentage score. Depending on which US state you're trying to gain certification in, candidates must score a 70% or 80% to pass the written exam. Also, you must score a 70% or 80% on the practical skills exam. Further, in your practical skills test, you must pass all **critical skills** components of the practical skills exam (such as handwashing, safety, and infection control), or you will automatically fail. If a candidate fails the practical skills exam, they will be provided with numerical codes that allow them to see where in the skills test they made any mistakes.

Scores usually are provided on the day of the test, but if a large number of test-takers are present at your test, your scores might be delivered the following day. Frequently, they are available online and via email. Licenses are mailed out to candidates who pass, and license registries (where you'll be listed if you pass your tests) are updated in the licensing system typically within 30 days. Approximately 18 states are part of the NNAAP registry, which streamlines the tests, having all proctored tests occurring at a designated proctor site

and administered by Pearson VUE or Prometric usually. These sites provide scores and a printout immediately after taking the test. The remaining 32 states handle their testing internally, and reporting will vary.

You can only take the test 3 times in 2 years following your training program. After the third time, you must repeat the training program before you can test again.

THE PRACTICAL SKILLS EXAM

The Practical Skills Exam is equally weighted in comparison to the written skills exam. Both the CNA and HHA exam require a practical skills exam, which consists of randomly selected skills, usually 3-6 skills, with handwashing always being one of the skills. The practical skills test is completed in 25-30 minutes (time limits vary by state). Possible skills used vary greatly and are based on real-life scenarios. Make sure you use your training time in class to practice any skills that you find difficult.

The following are the most commonly tested skills on the most popular CNA exams:

Commonly Tested Skills

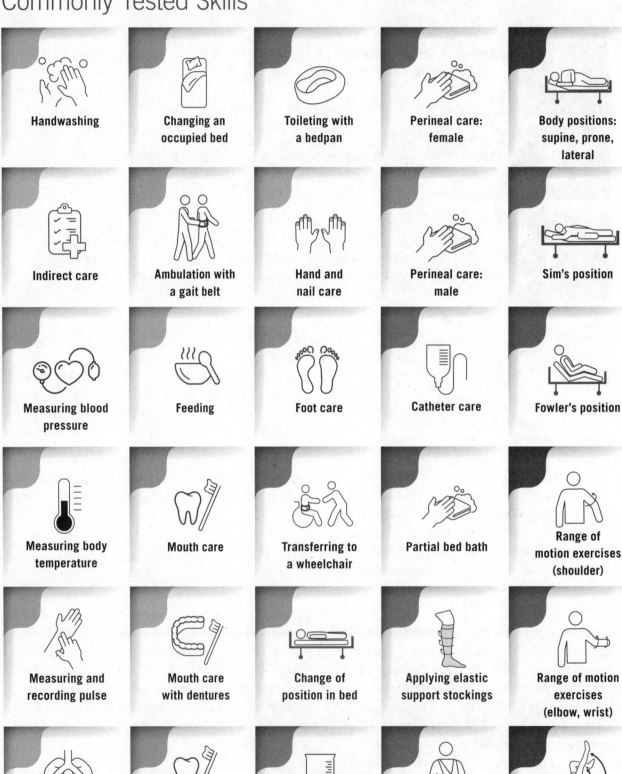

Handwashing

Changing an occupied bed

Toileting with a bedpan

Perineal care: female

Body positions: supine, prone, lateral

Indirect care

Ambulation with a gait belt

Hand and nail care

Perineal care: male

Sim's position

Measuring blood pressure

Feeding

Foot care

Catheter care

Fowler's position

Measuring body temperature

Mouth care

Transferring to a wheelchair

Partial bed bath

Range of motion exercises (shoulder)

Measuring and recording pulse

Mouth care with dentures

Change of position in bed

Applying elastic support stockings

Range of motion exercises (elbow, wrist)

Measuring and recording respiration

Mouth care for an unconscious patient

Measuring the output from a urinary bag

Dressing a resident with a weak arm

Range of motion exercises (hip, knee, ankle)

Most testing centers require you to provide your own volunteer for the practical skills exam. One solution is to schedule the exam back to back with another CNA/HHA candidate.

Each skill is rated based on a prescribed order set that is taught during the accredited program. Every misstep is docked; however, the candidate can announce an error as soon as they note it (for example, forgot to lock wheelchair, etc.), and they will receive partial credit for the error. In addition, handwashing is only done physically as the first skill. The candidate is then instructed to simply announce when they would wash their hands during each skillset.

Whichever CNA certification exam you take, each exam is always made up of two sections: the written examination, usually taken by computer, and the practical skills test, performed in front of a test evaluator. Depending on the certification requirements of your state, both tests typically require a score of 70-80% or better to pass. Always remember to check the requirements set out by your state to accurately prepare for your unique exam.

TESTING LOGISTICS

Now that we have covered the structure of the exam, the topics, and the scoring for both the written and practical skills tests, this final section is dedicated to testing logistics.

This includes the following:

- Scheduling
- Test Day
- Next Steps

Scheduling

We have already reviewed who can take the CNA and HHA exams and the requirements for an approved training program prior to testing. In addition, different states have specific preferences for testing. The three options are:

Pearson VUE—This national proctoring company works with 18 states and 2 territories to provide all CNA/HHA testing. This is external from the training program, and scheduling must be done independently from your program. The following link provides state-based information for scheduling: **https://home. pearsonvue.com/nurseaides**

Prometric—This national proctoring company is contracted to provide CNA/HHA testing in 13 states. The following link provides more information on the states covered and how to schedule: **https://www.prometric. com/test-takers/search/nurse-aide/select-state**

Correct handwashing is a non-negotiable. If you fail this section FOR ANY REASON (even if your error is how long you washed your hands), you will automatically fail, and your test will be stopped. Practice correct handwashing until it becomes second nature.

The exam itself costs approximately $100 for both components (written and practical skills tests) but will vary from state to state. In addition, your training program can help you fill out the paperwork required to verify you graduated from an approved training program. **You have only 24 months to take and pass the exam after graduation.** If you delay, you will have to retake the entire training program before you can take the exam.

Proctor at Training Site—Different states have different requirements around letting proctors come to the training site to complete large-scale testing for an entire graduating class. Many states offer this, and most CNA programs will offer this for their graduates to help ensure they can use the equipment and the setup they have practiced with during their practical skills test, thus increasing the likelihood of passing.

Test Day

Once you have scheduled your exam, it is important to prepare for the actual day of the test. Although you have no doubt spent time studying through this guide and the practice tests provided, there are a few things to remember for day-of logistics that will help you feel not only well-prepared but ready to go.

- **Get rest:** It may seem obvious that sleep should be the most important prerequisite the night before the exam. However, you may feel pressure to squeeze in one last study session the night before the test. This approach is a very unproductive one as it deprives you of much-needed sleep, which can lead to lower scores.

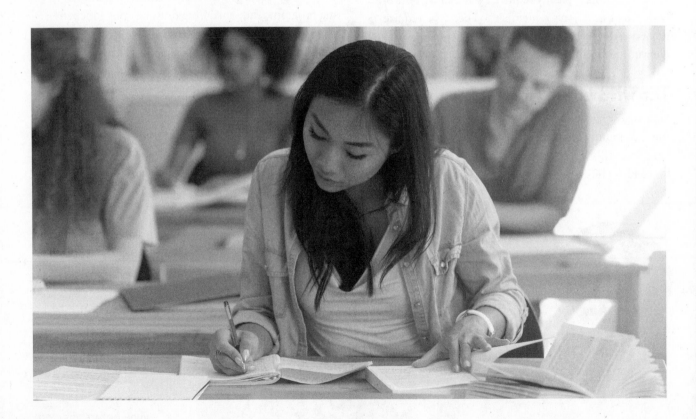

- **Wear comfortable clothing:** Scrubs are preferred as you will be required to wear these in the workplace. Wear layers that allow you to adjust easily based on the temperature of the testing room. Being too hot or too cold can prove distracting and decrease your score. **Avoid extra jewelry or add-on pieces.** Some testing locations have restrictions on jewelry outside of a wedding ring.

- **Leave early and block off time:** The CNA/HHA written exam itself is 90 minutes, and the practical skills exam is 30 minutes. However, with instructions and scheduled breaks, it works out to be approximately 2.5 hours. Plan to be there the entire day, avoiding any commitments beyond the exam. This will allow you to be fully present without worry about other appointments, work shifts, etc. In addition, this allows for any possible technical difficulties or other delays that may prolong the actual exam process.

- **Admit errors during Practical Skills testing if needed:** Every error is counted against you during your practical skills exam. However, admitting an error or oversight will provide you with partial credit. Do not feel bad or embarrassed to identify a known error or oversight. You deserve partial credit, and not announcing it may distract you and cause you to make additional mistakes.

NEXT STEPS

After you have passed your CNA/HHA exam, you are ready to look for employment within the medical field! Although it may take up to 30 days for your information to be updated and visible within the state licensure database, your printed test results can often be used when applying for employment.

- **License Terms:** Remember, your CNA/HHA license is only issued for two years. You will need to renew it (usually for free, but varies by state) every two years as long as you are working in the field. If you leave the field, you can still renew it every two years with proper continuing education. If you allow your license to lapse, you will have to take the training program again.

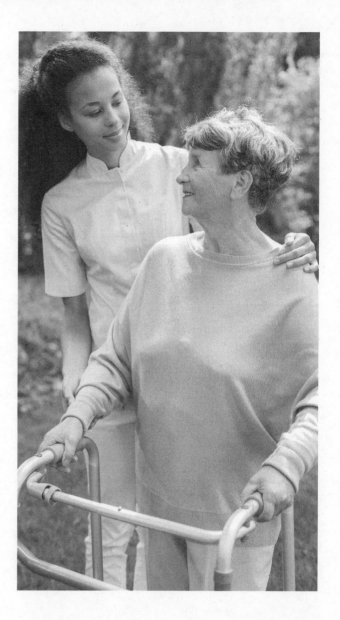

- **Reciprocity:** If you move to another state, your CNA/HHA license may or may not be accepted depending on the reciprocity rules and the training and clinical hours needed by the new state. For example, Colorado requires only 75 training hours and 16 clinical hours, but California requires 150 training hours and 100 clinical hours. Check with your new state to find out if reciprocity from your old state is possible. If not, you will have to take additional classes or complete a new training program to continue as a CNA/HHA.

PART II
PRE-TEST

2 | Finding Strengths and Weaknesses

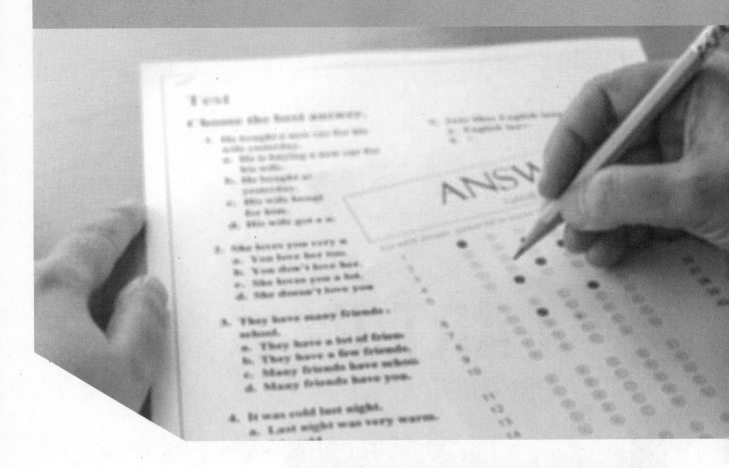

PRE-TEST

This pre-test is designed to help you recognize your strengths and weaknesses. The test questions cover information across some of the most common categories and subcategories presented on typical CNA and HHA exams.

CNA/HHA PRE-TEST ANSWER SHEET

1. Ⓐ Ⓑ Ⓒ Ⓓ   6. Ⓐ Ⓑ Ⓒ Ⓓ   11. Ⓐ Ⓑ Ⓒ Ⓓ   16. Ⓐ Ⓑ Ⓒ Ⓓ

2. Ⓐ Ⓑ Ⓒ Ⓓ   7. Ⓐ Ⓑ Ⓒ Ⓓ   12. Ⓐ Ⓑ Ⓒ Ⓓ   17. Ⓐ Ⓑ Ⓒ Ⓓ

3. Ⓐ Ⓑ Ⓒ Ⓓ   8. Ⓐ Ⓑ Ⓒ Ⓓ   13. Ⓐ Ⓑ Ⓒ Ⓓ   18. Ⓐ Ⓑ Ⓒ Ⓓ

4. Ⓐ Ⓑ Ⓒ Ⓓ   9. Ⓐ Ⓑ Ⓒ Ⓓ   14. Ⓐ Ⓑ Ⓒ Ⓓ   19. Ⓐ Ⓑ Ⓒ Ⓓ

5. Ⓐ Ⓑ Ⓒ Ⓓ   10. Ⓐ Ⓑ Ⓒ Ⓓ   15. Ⓐ Ⓑ Ⓒ Ⓓ   20. Ⓐ Ⓑ Ⓒ Ⓓ

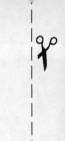

CNA/HHA PRE-TEST

30 minutes—20 questions

> **Directions:** Read each question below and choose the correct answer from the four choices provided. Only one choice is correct, so choose carefully.

1. According to the Center for Disease Control (CDC), the leading cause of death in adults older than 65 years is
   A. cancer.
   B. accidents.
   C. respiratory disease.
   D. coronary artery disease.

2. A nurse's aide should notify the nurse when the resident has a weight gain or loss of
   A. 0-1 lb.
   B. 1-2 lbs.
   C. 2-3 lbs.
   D. 3-5 lbs.

3. When helping a resident with a bedpan, the nurse's aide should
   A. remove the protective pads.
   B. allow the patient to be self-sufficient.
   C. examine under the covers as the patient is going to the bathroom to ensure accuracy.
   D. raise the head of the bed to a 90° angle.

4. The best way for nurse aides to get to know residents well in a long-term care facility is to
   A. ask them personal questions.
   B. discover their nonverbal communication style.
   C. find something they might like to do.
   D. bring in their favorite treats.

5. If a resident is gasping for air, then they are experiencing
   A. CAD.
   B. Pleura.
   C. BP.
   D. SOB.

6. One range of motion exercise for the ankle is
   A. plantar flexion.
   B. glute kicks.
   C. T-raises.
   D. weightless bicep curl.

7. To help an Islamic female patient honor her religious beliefs, she must be free to wear her
   A. frock coat.
   B. hijab.
   C. saffron.
   D. rosary beads.

8. Having a low-fiber and high-fat diet, drinking little water, and having a sedentary lifestyle can lead to
   A. constipation.
   B. frequent bowel movements.
   C. fast metabolism.
   D. hydration.

9. A living will is a legal document that offers patients

   A. end-of-life decisions ahead of time.

   B. the medical care they prefer or do not desire.

   C. identifiable health information to be kept private.

   D. the explanation of how patients should be treated.

10. If the physician order states "eat PO" in the patient's chart, then the meal is given

   A. post-operative.

   B. by mouth.

   C. pre-operative.

   D. when necessary.

11. A patient who has an extreme life experience or stressor that they cannot cope with is

   A. peaceful.

   B. displaced.

   C. in regression.

   D. in crisis.

12. Actively listening to a resident is important because it

   A. gives the aide the opportunity to plan a reaction.

   B. removes the need to ask questions.

   C. is the easiest thing to do.

   D. avoids misinterpretations.

13. Sterilization is the process of

   A. killing certain bacteria and viruses from surfaces.

   B. killing all germs.

   C. eliminating harmful germs.

   D. reducing harmful germs.

14. A patient who has just had a baby and is experiencing a sadness that does not go away most likely has

   A. postpartum depression.

   B. seasonal affective disorder.

   C. bipolar disorder.

   D. mania.

15. It is not within the nurse's aide scope of practice to

   A. share the contents of a patient's chart or record with the family.

   B. assist the nurse with delivering care.

   C. assist the patient with taking medication.

   D. share patient information with the next shift's staff.

16. The product used to promote the body's own immune system to defend a person against infection or disease is a(n)

   A. antibody.

   B. vaccine.

   C. antibiotic.

   D. steroid ointment.

17. The mechanical machine that lifts patients off the bed is called the

   A. Hoyer lift.

   B. chair lift.

   C. dumb waiter.

   D. manual sling.

18. A safety measure NOT used to prevent burns from hot liquids is to

   A. fill the patient's cup to the top.

   B. add ice.

   C. place a lid on the cup.

   D. help a patient who needs assistance with the hot drink.

19. After a blind patient settles into their room, it is important to never

    A. say your name when coming into the room.

    B. leave the door open.

    C. reorganize the furniture.

    D. mention where you place vital items, like food, in the room.

20. All of these are common examples of a CNA's and HHA's roles to foster independence in a resident EXCEPT:

    A. Offering choices and asking them for their opinions

    B. Encouraging participation in all outdoor activities

    C. Offering card games and reading materials in the communal area

    D. Encouraging them to do little things

ANSWER KEY AND EXPLANATIONS

1. D	**6.** A	**11.** D	**16.** B
2. D	**7.** B	**12.** D	**17.** A
3. D	**8.** A	**13.** B	**18.** A
4. B	**9.** B	**14.** A	**19.** C
5. D	**10.** B	**15.** A	**20.** B

1. **The correct answer is D.** According to the Center for Disease Control (CDC), coronary artery disease remains the leading cause of death in adults older than 65 years. The CDC also reports that cancer (choice A), accidents (choice B), and respiratory disease (choice C) are the second, third, and fourth leading causes of death, respectively, in adults older than 65 years.

2. **The correct answer is D.** If a resident has a weight gain or loss of 3-5 lbs., the nurse needs to be notified. A weight gain or loss of 0-1 lb. (choice A), 1-2 lbs. (choice B), or 2-3 lbs. (choice C) does not need to be reported to the nurse right away.

3. **The correct answer is D.** Raising the head of the bed to a 90° angle will allow the patient to be accommodated in a more natural position. Removing the protective pads (choice A) runs the risk of soiling the bed linens. Allowing the patient to be self-sufficient (choice B) may promote soiling accidents. Examining under the covers as the patient is going to the bathroom to ensure accuracy (choice C) denies the patient their dignity.

4. **The correct answer is B.** In working with a resident in a long-term care facility, discovering their nonverbal communication style, in response to different situations, can help a nurse aide interpret the resident's moods. Asking them personal questions (choice A) can overwhelm a resident and make them uncomfortable. Finding something they might like to do (choice C) and bringing in their favorite treats (choice D) may not help determine their personal style of communication.

5. **The correct answer is D.** A resident with SOB, shortness of breath, is gasping for air. A resident experiencing CAD (choice A) has coronary artery disease. Pleura (choice B) is the thin covering that protects the lungs. BP (choice C) is known as blood pressure.

6. **The correct answer is A.** Plantar flexion is an ankle exercise where toes are pushed downward and heels go up. Glute kicks (choice B) are used as a knee range of motion exercise. T-raises (choice C) are used as a shoulder range of motion exercise. Weightless bicep curls (choice D) are used as an elbow range of motion exercise.

7. **The correct answer is B.** Islamic women wear a hijab to honor and respect their submission to God. Hasidic Jewish men wear a frock coat (choice A) on special occasions. Buddhist men wear a saffron (choice C) to signify simplicity and detachment from materialism. Catholic Christians use rosary beads (choice D) sometimes when reciting the Rosary prayer.

8. **The correct answer is A.** Constipation is infrequent and difficult bowel movements that can be a result of a low-fiber and high-fat diet, drinking little water, and a having a sedentary lifestyle. Frequent bowel movements (choice B), fast metabolism (choice C), and hydration (choice D) are signs of a healthy digestive system.

9. **The correct answer is B.** Medical decisions that are preferred or not desired by the patient can be written in a living will. An advance directive (choice A) is a legal document indicating end-of-life decisions ahead of time. Protected Health Information (PHI) is identifiable health information that is required to be kept private (choice C) under the HIPAA law. The explanation of how patients should be treated (choice D) is expressed through the residents' rights.

10. **The correct answer is B.** In Latin, *per os* (abbreviated PO) means "by mouth." Post-operative (choice A) is written as "post- op" in the patient's chart. Pre-operative (choice C) is written as "pre-op" in a patient's chart. PRN (from the Latin term *pro re nata*) in the patient's chart is the acronym written for "when necessary" (choice D).

11. **The correct answer is D.** A crisis is a crucial situation or stressor that a patient has an overwhelming emotional response to for a period of time. A peaceful (choice A) patient is free from any conflict. A displaced (choice B) patient is forced out of their original position into another. A patient in regression (choice C) is moving towards a lesser condition.

12. **The correct answer is D.** Active listening allows the aide to concentrate on what is being said and avoid any misinterpretations. If the aide is actively listening, then the aide might not have the opportunity to plan a reaction (choice A). After actively listening, the aide will most likely need to ask questions (choice B) to make sure all the information that was heard is correct. Active listening is not the easiest thing to do (choice C), as it requires concentration and practice.

13. **The correct answer is B.** Killing all germs can only be achieved by sterilization. Disinfecting is the process of killing certain bacteria and viruses from surfaces (choice A), the process of eliminating (choice C) and reducing (choice D) harmful germs.

14. **The correct answer is A.** Women can experience postpartum depression after having a baby for many reasons. Seasonal affective disorder (choice A) is depression that occurs in a seasonal pattern, especially in the winter. Bipolar disorder (choice C) is having both manic and depressive moods. Mania (choice D) is an intense elevated mood or having extreme energy.

15. **The correct answer is A.** A nurse's aide cannot share the contents of a patient's chart or record with the family; it is the role of the doctor or nurse to do this. Assisting the nurse with delivering care (choice B), assisting the patient with taking medication (choice C), and sharing patient information

with the next shift's staff (choice D) are all part of a nurse aide's scope of practice.

16. **The correct answer is B.** Vaccines stimulate the body's own immune system to defend a person against infection or disease. Antibodies (choice A) are proteins produced by the body's immune system when it receives harmful antigens. Antibiotics (choice C) fight to kill microbes in or on the body. Steroid ointments (choice D) are topical agents used to treat inflammatory conditions, usually of the skin.

17. **The correct answer is A.** A Hoyer lift mechanically raises a patient off the bed. A chair lift (choice B) allows a patient to go up and down the stairs. A dumb waiter (choice C) is a small manual elevator that allows patients to move laundry or meals up and down floors. A manual sling (choice D) has a lifting device to assist, but the patient is lifted manually by another person.

18. **The correct answer is A.** It is not a good idea to fill the patient's cup to the top when trying to prevent burns from hot liquids. Adding ice (choice B), placing a lid on the cup (choice C), and helping a patient with the hot drink (choice D) are all safety measures used to prevent burns.

19. **The correct answer is C.** It is important to never reorganize the furniture after a blind patient settles in because doing so can cause the patient to fall. Saying your name when coming into the room (choice A), leaving the door open (choice B), and mentioning where you place vital items, like food, in the room (choice D) are important to a blind patient who is settling into their room.

20. **The correct answer is B.** Although light exercise is always helpful for an ambulatory resident, encouraging participation in all outdoor activities can be high-risk. Offering choices and asking them for their opinions (choice A), offering card games and reading materials in the communal area (choice C), and encouraging them to do little things (choice D), like combing their hair, can help to foster a resident's independence.

PART III
CNA & HHA REVIEW

FOUNDATIONS

HUMAN BODY BASICS

The foundational knowledge for every topic connected to being a well-trained Certified Nursing Assistant (CNA) or Home Health Aide (HHA) must begin with a solid understanding of the body through anatomy, physiology, and medical terminology. Learning the basics of the human body and its function, together with the most frequently used terms, will help you readily translate orders on a patient's chart without assistance during daily cares.

This chapter will give an overview of six major body systems that a CNA or HHA will encounter, how those systems work, and the terms associated with them. The following topics will be covered:

- Basic Anatomy
- Body Systems

- Musculoskeletal System
- Nervous System
- Circulatory and Respiratory Systems
- Digestive System
- Endocrine System
- Medical Terminology
  - Medication Management and Biology
  - Daily Cares
  - Therapies/Body Mechanics
  - Body Systems

BASIC ANATOMY

The human body is made up of many parts that work together to keep you alive. **Anatomy** is the study of the body and the organs, tissues, and cells within it. Having an awareness of the different parts of the body and where they are located is crucial to understanding how they work, which is also referred to as **physiology**.

Let's take a closer look at the basic components of every human body, including cells, tissues, and organs.

- **Tissues**—Tissues are groups of similar, specialized cells that function together as a unit and have similar structure and function. Organs are made of tissues. One example is lung tissue, which is made up of lung cells. The following graphic indicates other tissue types and their locations in the body.

Types of Tissues

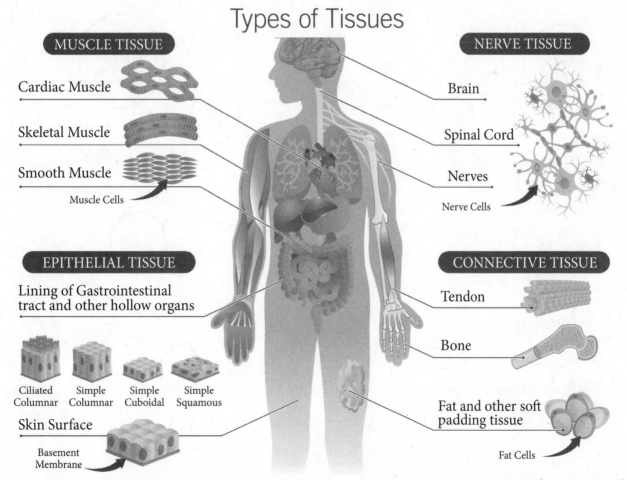

MUSCLE TISSUE
- Cardiac Muscle
- Skeletal Muscle
- Smooth Muscle

Muscle Cells

NERVE TISSUE
- Brain
- Spinal Cord
- Nerves

Nerve Cells

EPITHELIAL TISSUE
Lining of Gastrointestinal tract and other hollow organs

Ciliated Columnar   Simple Columnar   Simple Cuboidal   Simple Squamous

Skin Surface

Basement Membrane

CONNECTIVE TISSUE
- Tendon
- Bone
- Fat and other soft padding tissue

Fat Cells

Skin is also an organ.

Common Cell Types

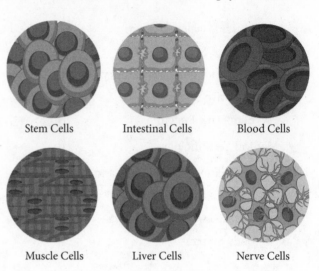

- **Cells**—Cells are the basic building blocks of our bodies. Everything in our bodies is made up of cells. There are numerous types of cells in your body, each specifically created to work in a distinctive way to keep you alive. Common examples of these cells are blood cells and lung cells. The image to the right shows some other common cell types.

- **Organs**—Organs are groups of tissues that complete a specialized function in the body. Examples include the brain, kidneys, stomach, skin, and lungs. The following graphic reviews the primary internal organs.

Internal Organs

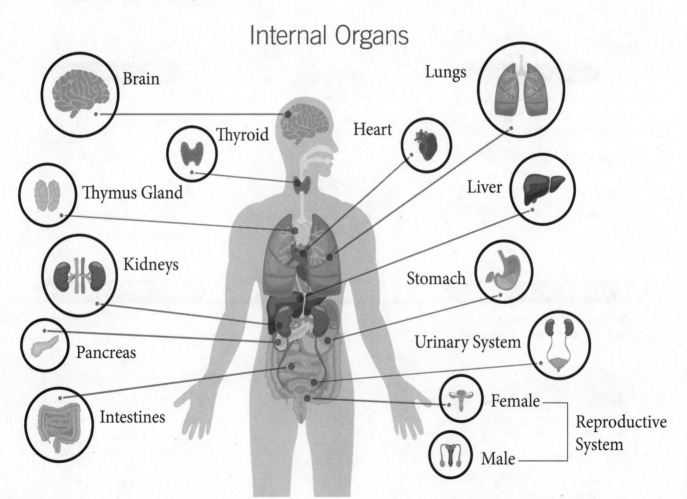

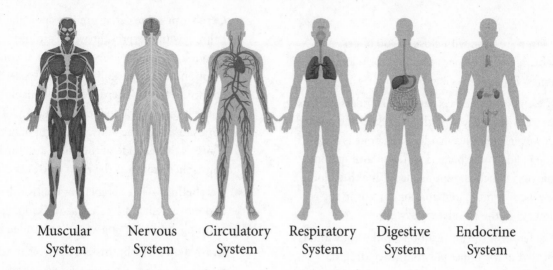

| Muscular System | Nervous System | Circulatory System | Respiratory System | Digestive System | Endocrine System |

BODY SYSTEMS

Now that we have reviewed the basic building blocks of the human body, we can explore how everything works together to keep you alive. Organs work together in systems that have specific functions. Although organs may be present in more than one system, they have a primary function that is connected to one of the **body systems**.

There is a total of 12-14 body systems (depending on how they are grouped), but seven encompass the majority of all complications and cares a CNA or HHA may encounter. However, in this chapter, we will not focus on the reproductive system, as it generally falls outside of the scope of the duties expected of a CNA or HHA. The following six systems are most relevant to a CNA or HHA:

- Musculoskeletal System
- Nervous System
- Circulatory System
- Respiratory System
- Digestive System
- Endocrine System

Musculoskeletal System

The **musculoskeletal system** is a combination of the muscles and bones within the human body. There are over 400 muscles and 206 bones in the adult body. There are almost 300 bones in an infant's body, but many fuse by adulthood. The main function of this system is to provide structure and strength for the body. Without a skeleton, humans would not be able to stand, walk, eat, or climb. If you think about animals without a skeleton (such as a jellyfish), you can see how important the skeleton is to structure and movement in the human body. Muscles complement the bones, giving flexibility and strength to the body. Where bones give you form and allow you to stand, it is the muscle connected to the bone that allows you to move, bend, jump, and generally change position with ease.

Here is more information about each component of the musculoskeletal system:

Muscles

There are 3 types of **muscles**—skeletal, smooth, and cardiac.

- **Skeletal Muscles**—These muscles are attached to bones by tendons. They are the muscles directly related to your movement and strength.
- **Smooth Muscles**—These muscles are found inside the walls of hollow organs, such as the stomach, intestines, and uterus. The most common smooth muscle is found in the digestive system and is responsible for moving food through the gastrointestinal tract.
- **Cardiac Muscle**—This muscle is located in the heart and is responsible for pumping blood throughout the body.

Bones

- Infants are born with close to 300 bones. As babies grow, the bones fuse and form longer bones. An adult has 206 bones.

- The anatomy of bones can be misunderstood, as they are generally thought of as hard and sturdy. However, only the outside of the bone is hard. The inside of the bone is soft, containing bone marrow, which is responsible for making blood. We'll cover more information on this in the section about the circulatory system.

- The femur is the longest bone in the body and is located in the upper part of the leg (thigh).

- The 3 smallest bones in the body are all located in the ear: the malleus, incus, and stapes. The stapes is technically the smallest bone in the body.

Nervous System

The **nervous system** is the control center of the body. It is responsible for interpreting data from the sensory organs via nerves, which travel through the spinal cord and are processed in the brain. The nervous system controls all aspects of the body, including autonomic and somatic body processes. **Autonomic** body processes happen automatically without you having to think about it, such as breathing. **Somatic** body processes are voluntary and require conscious thought, such as walking and talking.

Once messages span off from the spinal cord, they travel through the **Peripheral Nervous System**. The illustration to the right helps to provide a visual of this system.

The brain and spinal cord make up the **Central Nervous System** (CNS). The following covers the two main components of the CNS.

The Brain

The **brain** is the control center of your body. Your brain sends constant messages throughout your body to ensure that your body functions and remains healthy.

There are three major parts to the brain, the **cerebrum**, **cerebellum**, and **brainstem**. The brain image shown to the right identifies where these parts are located within the brain.

- **Cerebrum**—The cerebrum is responsible for helping you interpret the world around you through the use of your five senses. It controls emotions and your ability to read, speak, learn, and think freely. There are two hemispheres in the brain—right and left—that control the opposite side of the body. The right hemisphere controls the left side of the body, and the left hemisphere controls the right side of the body.

- **Cerebellum**—The cerebellum controls balance and movement. Tasks such as walking, dancing, running, and climbing are all controlled here.

- **Brainstem**—The brainstem controls the autonomic, or automatic, activities your body does without you thinking about them. This includes breathing, heart pumping, and blinking.

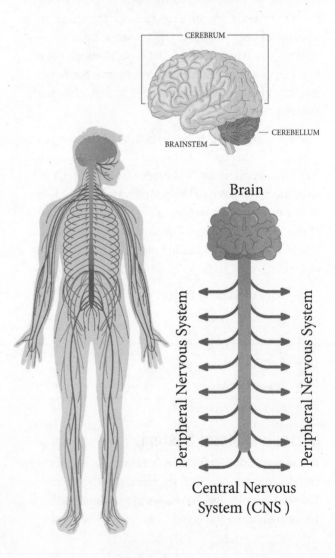

Spinal Cord

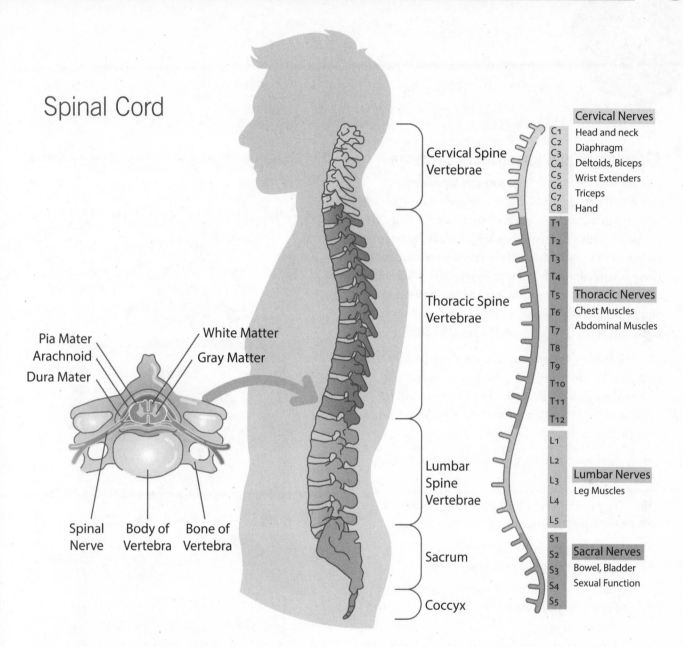

C1	**Cervical Nerves**
C2	Head and neck
C3	Diaphragm
C4	Deltoids, Biceps
C5	Wrist Extenders
C6	Triceps
C7	Hand
C8	

Cervical Spine Vertebrae

Thoracic Spine Vertebrae

Lumbar Spine Vertebrae

Sacrum

Coccyx

Pia Mater
Arachnoid
Dura Mater

White Matter
Gray Matter

Spinal Nerve
Body of Vertebra
Bone of Vertebra

Thoracic Nerves
Chest Muscles
Abdominal Muscles

Lumbar Nerves
Leg Muscles

Sacral Nerves
Bowel, Bladder
Sexual Function

The Spinal Cord

The **spinal cord** runs down your back from the brainstem to the tailbone. It is protected by 33 bones in your back called **vertebrae**, which are a series of small bones interlocked to each other, each with a spinal canal that the spinal cord runs through. This design allows for maximum protection of the spinal cord from injury while also providing free range of motion for the person. If the vertebrae were simply one solid bone, bending over, twisting, and other similar movements would be impossible.

The image above shows the different sections of the spinal cord as well as the inside of a vertebra.

Nerves

Similar in structure to a bundle of wires or cables, **nerves** (formed by cells called neurons) are responsible for delivering every message your brain sends. They run throughout every single part of your body, from your heart to your fingertips. They both deliver messages from the brain (such as a message to lift your leg to avoid tripping) and to the brain (such as a pain message when your leg hits the stairs).

Capillaries are small blood vessels that can carry both oxygenated and deoxygenated blood. They can be found, for example, in your hands and feet.

Circulatory and Respiratory Systems

The **circulatory system** is responsible for both the delivery of nutrients and oxygen and the removal of waste (such as carbon dioxide) throughout the body via the blood. This system overlaps with the **cardiovascular system**, and some texts use these terms interchangeably. Every cell in your body requires oxygen and other nutrients. Your circulatory system is made up of thousands of miles of blood vessels of varying sizes that allow it to easily transport things to even the smallest cells.

The **respiratory system** works in conjunction with the circulatory system, providing oxygen and expelling carbon dioxide from the body. The main parts of the circulatory and respiratory systems are the heart, lungs, trachea, blood, and blood vessels.

The cycle of the circulatory and respiratory systems is as follows:

1. The person takes a breath, causing oxygen to flow down the trachea and into the lungs.

2. The lungs transfer the oxygen in **alveoli**, tiny sacs throughout the lung tissue.

3. Red blood cells pick up the oxygen and carry it to cells that need oxygen via blood vessels called **arteries**.

4. The heart pumps the blood, moving the red blood cells to their destination.

5. After delivering the oxygen, the red blood cells pick up carbon dioxide (waste) and travel back to the lungs via blood vessels called **veins**.

6. The lungs exhale the carbon dioxide waste, and the process starts all over again.

The following illustration shows how all the parts work together:

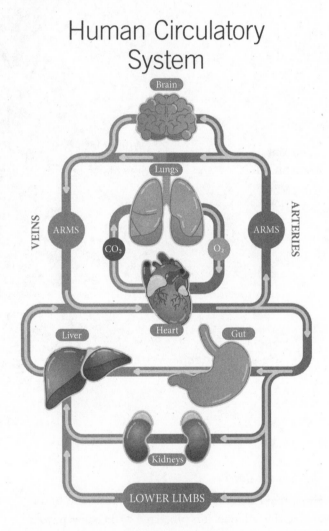

The following are important parts that make up the circulatory and respiratory systems:

- **Blood**—The average adult body is made up of 5 to 7 quarts of blood. Blood production occurs in the bone marrow and is then distributed into the bloodstream. Blood is composed of 4 parts:

○ **Red Blood Cells**—Red blood cells (RBCs) are the heaviest and most plentiful blood cell present in the blood. They are what give blood a red color and are responsible for carrying and delivering oxygen and removing carbon dioxide from the body. They make up 35-48% of blood composition.

○ **White Blood Cells**—White blood cells (WBCs) are much larger in size in comparison to red blood cells, although you have far fewer of them. They are responsible for fighting off infections and are often referred to as the "body's army." When your body detects an infection, white blood cell production increases dramatically to combat it quickly and efficiently. WBCs make up less than 1% of your blood during times of good health.

○ **Platelets**—Platelets are responsible for clotting the blood and repairing tissue damage. When blood vessels are damaged, such as through an injury, platelets activate and form a wall to stop the bleeding, and this process is referred to as clotting. They then work to repair the damage. They also make up less than 1% of your blood.

○ **Plasma**—Plasma is the liquid that contains all the blood components mentioned above.

Without plasma, RBCs, WBCs, and platelets could not move through the body to complete their jobs. Plasma makes up approximately half of your blood composition.

● **The Heart**—The heart is a muscle that is responsible for pumping blood. It operates through electrical pulses that cause it to beat rhythmically, pumping blood both to the body with life-giving oxygen and up to the lungs with carbon dioxide waste. The heart is controlled via the brainstem and pumps autonomously without the person thinking about it. When the heart suddenly stops beating, it is referred to as **cardiac arrest**, also called a heart attack. When the heart beats irregularly, it is called an **arrhythmia**. The heart is divided into two sides—one is responsible for pumping the oxygen-rich blood and the other for the carbon-dioxide filled blood.

● **The Lungs**—The lungs are composed of two identical organs that are responsible for breathing. They expand when air is inhaled and deflate as air is expelled. The inside of the lungs resembles small trees and are called **bronchi**. At the tissue level, small sacs called **alveoli** hold the oxygen and provide it to the red blood cells so they can transport it to the rest of the body.

Blood Structure

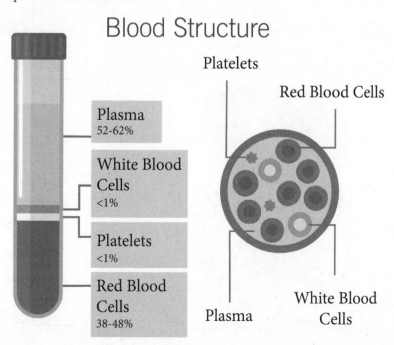

Plasma
52-62%

White Blood Cells
<1%

Platelets
<1%

Red Blood Cells
38-48%

Platelets

Red Blood Cells

Plasma

White Blood Cells

Digestive System

The **digestive system** is responsible for all food-related processes. This includes eating, digesting, absorbing the nutrients into the bloodstream, and excretion of waste. The digestive system starts with your mouth and ends with your anus. It provides all the energy your body needs to stay alive and function properly. The following is a 5-step guide to the digestive process:

Step 1: Ingestion—You take a bite of food and use your teeth and tongue to grind it into small pieces. Your saliva begins the digestive process by breaking down starch.

Step 2: Propulsion—You swallow the food, and it works its way down your esophagus through a muscle process called **peristalsis**.

Step 3: Digestion—The food enters the stomach, and enzymes and gastric acid begin to break down the food. The partially digested food, also called **chyme**, is then emptied into the duodenum. **Bile**, which is produced by the liver and stored in the gallbladder, is released into the duodenum to help break down fats in the food. The pancreas also releases enzymes to break down carbohydrates, proteins, and some fats. The food then moves into the small intestine.

Step 4: Absorption—The small intestine then absorbs important nutrients into the bloodstream. The food then enters the large intestine, or colon, which is responsible for absorbing water and vitamins, processing any undigested food (such as fiber), and storing waste before it is finally removed. On average, this part of digestion takes approximately 36 hours.

Step 5: Excretion—The final process is excretion, or removal of the waste. It slowly makes its way down the large intestine, with the rectum controlling whether it is time to release the waste or wait. Many factors affect this process, including hydration. The drier the food, the harder it is to move through the colon.

The following illustration shows the steps of the digestion process and where they occur in the digestive system:

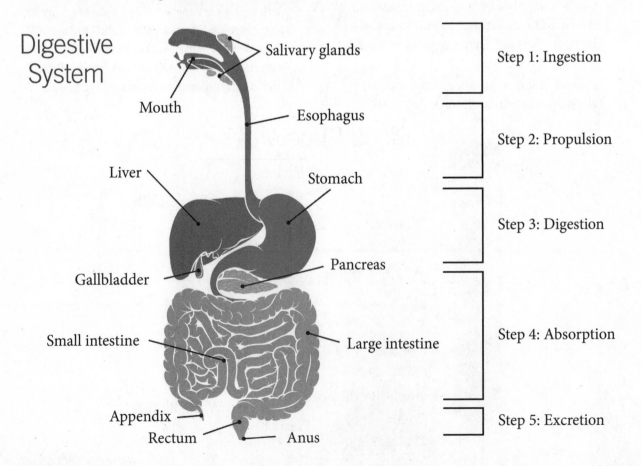

Endocrine System

The final system we will review is the **endocrine system**. Although this is one of the smaller systems, it is extremely important to understand for CNAs and HHAs as many patients you will interact with will have problems related to this system. The endocrine system is responsible for regulating hormones. This includes everything from insulin to estrogen and testosterone.

The following is a diagram of the endocrine system and its major components:

Endocrine System

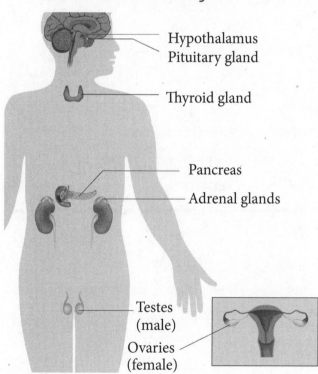

The following are important components related to the endocrine system:

- **The Hypothalamus and the Pituitary Gland**— Both located in the brain, these two glands work together to regulate the number of hormones released throughout the body. The **hypothalamus** is like a thermometer, keeping constant tabs on the levels of all hormones in the body.

The **pituitary gland** receives "orders" from the hypothalamus and acts as a director for the other endocrine glands and organs, sending out orders on necessary hormone adjustments.

- **Thyroid**—This gland is responsible for releasing hormones that control your **metabolism**. This directly correlates to your energy and how your body uses it.

- **Adrenal Glands**—These glands produce sex hormones (such as estrogen), adrenaline, and cortisol. **Cortisol** is a type of natural steroid that is produced in response to stresses, including blood sugar shifts and trauma, such as an accident or natural disaster.

- **Reproductive Organs**—This includes the ovaries and testes, both of which produce reproductive hormones including estrogen and testosterone.

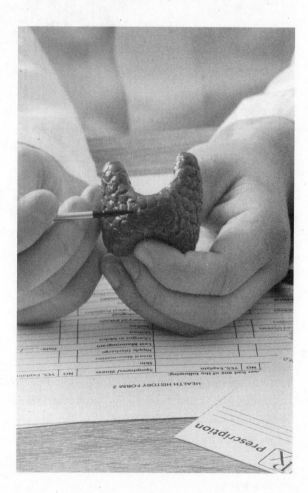

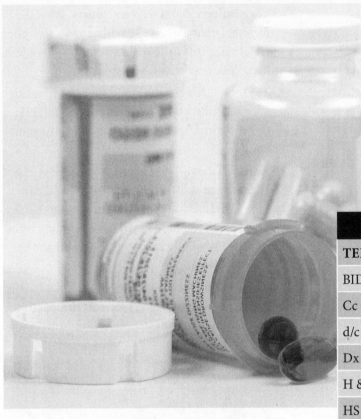

MEDICAL TERMINOLOGY

There is a great deal of medical terminology for CNAs and HHAs to memorize and be aware of to provide safe and proper care for their patients. Although it is impossible to memorize every possible term used in the medical field, it is important to know the basics. The next section of this chapter presents medical terminology that is focused on the most frequently used terms you'll encounter both in Activities of Daily Living (ADLs) and when talking about body systems.

Medication Management and Biology

Much of the medical terminology under this heading is related to frequency, duration, and amount of medication. This can be useful information if you do not completely understand the full term. For example *chole-* has to do with the gallbladder as noted in cholecystectomy, which is the removal of the gallbladder.

On the right is a list of common terms with definitions of each term.

COMMON TERMS	
TERM	**DEFINITION**
BID	Twice a day
Cc	Cubic centimeters
d/c	Discontinue
Dx	Diagnosis
H & P	History and Physical
HS	Hour of sleep; at bedtime
IV	Intravenous
Kardex	Quick reference card of medical needs
(Lt)	Left
LTC	Long-term care
mg	Milligram
ml	Milliliter
Occult	Hidden
O^2	Oxygen
per	By or through
Pt/pt	Patient
Q	Every
Q2/Q3 etc.	Every 2 hours, 3 hours, etc.
QID	Everyday
Sub Q	Subcutaneous
Via	By way of
Δ	Delta symbol = change

Daily Care

Much of the terminology related to your work as a CNA or HHA will fall under the heading of daily care. The terms below refer to the types of care you will perform and how to document those cares.

DAILY CARE TERMS	
TERM	DEFINITION
AMB	Ambulatory
PRN	As needed
AX	Axillary
inh	Inhaled
BM	Bowel movement
BP	Blood pressure
PO	By mouth
Centigrade	Metric unit of temperature
Fahrenheit	US unit of temperature
Emesis	Vomiting
HOB	Head of bed
HOH	Hard of hearing
I & O	Intake and output
Incontinence	Inability to control urine
Kg	Kilograms
lb	Pounds
w/c	Wheelchair
OOB	Out of bed
SOB	Shortness of breath
s/s	Signs and symptoms
TPR	Temperature, pulse, and respirations
NKA	No known allergies
NPO	Nothing by mouth
VS	Vital signs
Wt	Weight
Ht	Height

TERM	DEFINITION
AMT	Amount
Aspiration	Liquid and food getting into lungs
H_2O	Water
NCS	No concentrated sweets

Therapies and Body Mechanics

There are precise medical terms used in body mechanics and therapies. A lot of these have to do with positioning and the placement of the body, and it is often the CNA's or HHA's duty to help the patient complete daily therapeutic exercises.

THERAPIES & BODY TERMS	
TERM	DEFINITION
Abduction	Moving away from the body
Adduction	Moving towards the body
Anterior	Toward the front
Distal	Further from the torso
Dorsal	Top/Back
RT	Respiratory therapist
Extension	To extend
Flexion	To bend
PT	Physical therapist
Lateral	Away from midline of body
Medial	Towards midline of body
OT	Occupational therapist
Supine	Lying on back
Sims' Position	Lying on left side, right knee up
Fowler's Position	HOB is at 45 to 60 degrees
Proximal	Closer to the torso
Trendelenburg Position	HOB lower than feet
Prone	Lying face down

Body Systems

The bulk of the terms you will encounter on the job will, in some way, be related to the body and the systems within it. These terms refer to the part of the body they are connected to. For example, the term *colo-* relates to the colon, and the term *cranio-* relates to the skull.

BODY SYSTEMS TERMS	
TERM	**DEFINITION**
Acute	Sudden onset
Chronic	Long term
Edema	Swelling
ECG or EKG	Electrocardiogram
Cranio	Relating to the skull
Pelvic	Relating to the pelvis
Spinal	Relating to the back
Thoracic	Relating to the chest
Ventral	Relating to the abdomen
CAD	Coronary artery disease
CCU	Cardiac care unit
Ceph	Relating to the head
Chole	Relating to the gallbladder
Colo	Relating to the colon
Coronary	Relating to the heart
Embolus	A moving blood clot
Gastro	Relating to the stomach
Hepa	Relating to the liver
Neph	Relating to the kidney
Neuro	Relating to the nervous system/brain
Ortho	Relating to bones
Phleb	Relating to the veins
Pleural	Relating to the lungs

TERM	**DEFINITION**
Thrombus	A fixed blood clot
Uro	Relating to the urinary system
Vascular	Related to blood vessels
Unilateral	On one side
Bilateral	On both sides
Brady	Slow
Dys	Difficult or painful
Endo	Internal
Epi	On or over
Geri	Relating to the older, geriatric population
Heme/a	Related to blood
Intra	Within
Noc	Night
Peri	Around
Poly	Many

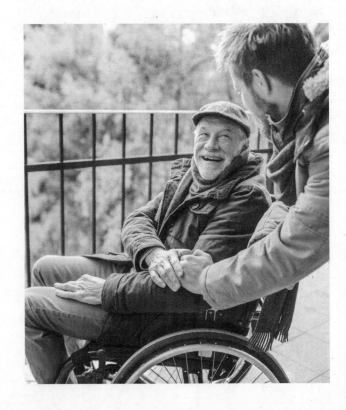

MINI-QUIZ: ANATOMY, PHYSIOLOGY, AND MEDICAL TERMINOLOGY

Directions: Read each question below and choose the correct answer from the four choices provided. Only one choice is correct, so choose carefully.

1. What are the names of the three types of muscle?

   A. Smooth, rough, cardiac

   B. Smooth, cardiac, skeletal

   C. Cardiac, internal, external

   D. Cardiac, skeletal, rough

2. How many bones are in an adult's body?

   A. Almost 300

   B. 216

   C. 270

   D. 206

3. The basic building blocks of the human body are called

   A. tissues.

   B. organs.

   C. cells.

   D. systems.

4. Red blood cells are responsible for

   A. transporting oxygen.

   B. fighting off infection.

   C. clotting.

   D. breathing.

5. The system responsible for regulating hormones is the _____system.

   A. digestive

   B. circulatory

   C. respiratory

   D. endocrine

6. Which system contains the duodenum?

   A. Musculoskeletal

   B. Digestive

   C. Endocrine

   D. Respiratory

7. Which part of the brain is responsible for controlling emotions?

   A. Cerebrum

   B. Cerebellum

   C. Brainstem

   D. Nerves

8. Which organ controls the production and release of insulin?

   A. Thyroid

   B. Liver

   C. Pancreas

   D. Thymus

9. Blood is made in which of the following locations?

   A. Heart

   B. Lungs

   C. Blood vessels

   D. Bone marrow

10. The central nervous system includes the

    A. brain.

    B. spinal cord.

    C. brain and the spinal cord.

    D. peripheral nerves.

11. A patient must take their medicine twice a day. Which of the following should you expect to see on the prescription?

    A. QID

    B. 2D

    C. BID

    D. 2x/day

12. A doctor states they are worried about their patient's hepatic levels. Which organ are they referring to?

    A. Liver

    B. Kidney

    C. Stomach

    D. Colon

13. The nurse asks you to track how much a patient drinks and voids. What is the abbreviation for this request?

    A. HOH

    B. I & O

    C. SOB

    D. OOB

14. A fine motor therapy is prescribed by a(n) _____ therapist.

    A. respiratory

    B. occupational

    C. speech

    D. physical

15. Which of the following terms means *slow*?

    A. Epi

    B. Noc

    C. Brady

    D. Via

16. Which of the following is the medical abbreviation for the metric unit for weight?

    A. cc

    B. ml

    C. lb.

    D. kg

17. If a patient only uses a medicated lotion as needed, the label on the bottle will say which of the following?

    A. PO

    B. PRN

    C. AN

    D. QID

18. A procedure that involves the blood will start with which of the following prefixes?

    A. Hema-

    B. Phleb-

    C. Endo-

    D. Ortho-

19. A patient needs to lie face down on the bed. What type of position is this?

    A. Supine

    B. Fowler's position

    C. Prone

    D. Trendelenburg position

20. A patient is set to have surgery in the morning, and the charge nurse asks if they have any allergies. When you check the chart, you see NKA. What type of allergy is documented?

    A. Sulfa

    B. Penicillin

    C. Codeine

    D. None

ANSWER KEY AND EXPLANATIONS

1. B	**5.** D	**9.** D	**13.** B	**17.** B
2. D	**6.** B	**10.** C	**14.** B	**18.** A
3. C	**7.** A	**11.** C	**15.** C	**19.** C
4. A	**8.** C	**12.** A	**16.** D	**20.** D

1. **The correct answer is B.** The three types of muscle are smooth (which are inside your body, such as the stomach), cardiac (in your heart), and skeletal (used for movement). There are no rough muscles (choices A and D). Also, muscles are not described as internal and external (choice C).

2. **The correct answer is D.** There are 206 bones in the adult body. An infant is born with almost 300 bones (choice A), and many fuse slowly over time (choices B and C). However, by adulthood, we have 206 distinct bones.

3. **The correct answer is C.** The basic building blocks of the human body are called cells. Tissues (choice A) are groups of specialized cells, and organs (choice B) are groups of specialized tissue. Body systems (choice D) are made up of organs.

4. **The correct answer is A.** Red blood cells are responsible for transporting and delivering oxygen. White blood cells fight off infection (choice B). Platelets are responsible for clotting (choice C). The lungs are responsible for breathing (choice D).

5. **The correct answer is D.** The endocrine system is responsible for regulating hormones. The digestive system (choice A) is responsible for food digestion and absorption. The circulatory system (choice B) is responsible for carrying oxygen and nutrients throughout the body. The respiratory system (choice C) is responsible for breathing.

6. **The correct answer is B.** The duodenum is in the digestive system in between the stomach and the small intestine. Choices A, C, and D are incorrect.

7. **The correct answer is A.** The cerebrum is responsible for controlling all input from your five senses and then interpreting it, and this includes emotions. The cerebellum (choice B) is responsible for balance and movement. The brainstem (choice C) is responsible for all autonomous or automatic functions like breathing or blinking. Nerves (choice D) simply carry messages back and forth to the brain.

8. **The correct answer is C.** The pancreas controls the production and release of insulin. The thyroid and thymus (choices A and D) are glands that control metabolism and T-cell production, respectively, not insulin. The liver (choice B) controls the production of bile, not insulin.

9. **The correct answer is D.** Blood is made in the bone marrow, which is the soft inside part of the bone. It is not made in the heart (choice A), the lungs (choice B), or the blood vessels (choice C).

10. **The correct answer is C.** The central nervous system (CNS) consists of the brain and the spinal cord. Choices A and B only include one part of the CNS. Peripheral nerves (choice D) are part of the peripheral nervous system (PNS) and not the central nervous system (CNS).

11. **The correct answer is C.** BID is the abbreviation for twice a day. QID (choice A) refers to every day. 2D (choice B) is not an acceptable term, and 2x/day (choice D) is not the accepted, medical way to write this frequency.

12. **The correct answer is A.** *Hepa-* is the root for terms related to the liver. A kidney (choice B) related term starts with *neph-*. A stomach (choice

C) related term starts with *gastro-*. A colon (choice D) related term starts with *colo-*.

13. **The correct answer is B.** I & O refers to intake and output, which is related to how much a patient drinks (and eats) and how much they void. HOH (choice A) stands for hard of hearing. SOB (choice C) stands for shortness of breath. OOB (choice D) stands for out of bed.

14. **The correct answer is B.** The occupational therapist is responsible for therapies that increase activities of daily living. This includes activities like feeding oneself or writing. A respiratory therapist (choice A) is responsible for breathing-related treatments. A speech therapist (choice C) is responsible for feeding and other oral therapies such as talking or swallowing. A physical therapist (choice D) is responsible for mobility and gross motor skills.

15. **The correct answer is C.** *Brady* refers to "slow," such as *bradycardia*, which means a slower than normal heartbeat. *Epi* (choice A) means "on or over." *Noc* (choice B) means "night." *Via* (choice D) means "through."

16. **The correct answer is D.** The medical abbreviation for the metric unit for weight is kg, which stands for kilogram. Cc (choice A) stands for cubic centimeter, and ml (choice B) stands for milliliter, both of which measure liquids. Lb. (choice C) stands for pound, which is the American unit for weight.

17. **The correct answer is B.** PRN is the official abbreviation for an "as needed" prescription. PO (choice A) means by mouth. AN (choice C) is not an official abbreviation. QID (choice D) means every day.

18. **The correct answer is A.** *Hema-* is the prefix related to blood. *Phleb-* (choice B) is related to veins specifically. *Endo-* (choice C) is related to internal medicine. *Ortho-* (choice D) is related to the bones.

19. **The correct answer is C.** *Prone* is the term for lying in a face down position. *Supine* (choice A) means lying on your back. Fowler's position (choice B) is when the head of the bed is at a 45-60 degree angle. A Trendelenburg position (choice D) is when the head of the bed is below the feet and is rarely ordered.

20. **The correct answer is D.** NKA stands for no known allergies. All other allergies would be documented by full name in the chart.

SUMMING IT UP

- Anatomy is the study of your body and the organs, tissues, and cells within it.

- Physiology is the awareness of the different parts of the body, where they are located, and how they work.

- The basic components of every human body are cells, tissues, and organs.

- CNAs and HHAs should be familiar with these six body systems: musculoskeletal system, nervous system, circulatory system, respiratory system, digestive system, and endocrine system.

  - The musculoskeletal system is a combination of the muscles and bones within the human body.

  - The nervous system is the control center of the body including the brain, spinal cord, and nerves.

  - The circulatory system is responsible for both the delivery of nutrients and oxygen and the removal of waste (such as carbon dioxide) throughout the body via the blood.

  - The respiratory system works in conjunction with the circulatory system, providing oxygen and expelling carbon dioxide from the body.

  - The digestive system is responsible for all food-related processes including eating, digesting, absorbing nutrients into the bloodstream, and excreting waste.

  - The endocrine system regulates hormones.

- There is a great deal of medical terminology for CNAs and HHAs to memorize to provide safe and proper care for their patients, including terms about medication management, patient biology, daily care, therapy, body mechanics, and body systems.

ROLES OF THE CNA & HHA

OVERVIEW

ROLES AND RESPONSIBILITIES

In this section, we will focus on an overview of the roles and responsibilities of a CNA and HHA. It is important to always make sure you act within your scope of practice, doing only what you were trained and licensed to do. If you are asked by someone to go outside your scope of practice in any way, it is important to tell the person it is outside your scope of practice and refuse to complete whatever tasks they've requested you do. Completing the tasks could cause you to lose your license.

Activities of Daily Living

The bulk of your work as a CNA or HHA encompasses Activities of Daily Living (ADLs). ADLs are vital to both the physical and mental health of residents in your care, and your skillset and the care you use when you provide them are of utmost importance. The following are the basic ADLs that fall within the role and responsibility of a CNA and HHA:

Feeding

As a CNA, you will help with feeding in many ways, from providing verbal cues to a memory-impaired resident to doing a full physical feeding for a quadriplegic resident.

Grooming

Grooming includes helping residents care for their hair, attach wigs, clean fingernails, shave, brush their teeth, place dentures, add requested jewelry and makeup, and more. Your job is to make sure the resident looks their best based on the guidance they and their family have provided.

Bathing

Residents are often placed on a bathing schedule, but they can also request a bath at any time. It is your responsibility to complete bathing in a safe and dignified manner. Most residents use a shower chair and will require a transfer. In addition, some facilities and homes have specialized bathtubs that may require the use of a Hoyer lift. Make sure to follow all safety protocols, including requesting help if necessary.

Dressing

It is the responsibility of the CNA to assist the resident in selecting appropriate clothes, getting dressed, and ensuring they have nonslip socks or shoes on.

Toileting

This includes both assistance on and off the commode as well as changing any sheets or undergarments as

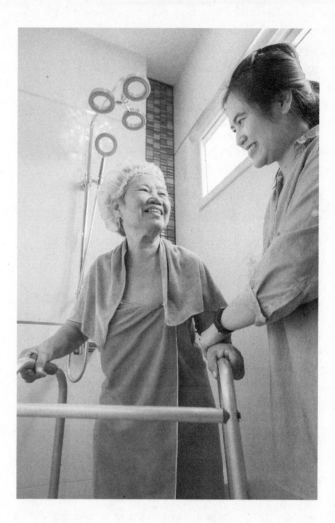

needed. For those that are incontinent, you are responsible for all perineal care (or pericare), which is cleaning the patient's external genitalia. Toileting also includes caring for patients with catheters in place.

Activities

Every facility has an activity calendar. It is within your role to announce the activities of the day and invite the resident to attend. You will then provide transportation within the facility if needed. In addition, CNAs and HHAs are encouraged to engage in one-on-one activities with patients as their schedule allows. This can include playing cards, reading the paper aloud, or even just conversing.

Medical Equipment and Assistance

A CNA is often asked to gather, prepare, and even sanitize necessary equipment for the nurse to use. At times, a CNA can also be required to help with the equipment. Nurses can delegate certain tasks to CNAs and HHAs, such as drawing blood, checking blood glucose levels, and obtaining EKGs, if the CNA has additional certifications for those tasks.

Common medical equipment and assistance areas for basic CNAs include the following:

- Assisting with catheter changes
- Assisting with blood draws
- Assisting with pressure ulcers and other wounds requiring dressings
- Putting on compression hoses/socks
- Sanitizing Hoyer lifts, catheter tools, cleaning tools, etc.

Always be aware of your scope of practice when assisting. If you are concerned that the task goes outside of your practice as a CNA, speak up immediately. Patient safety is the priority.

Vital Signs and Daily Observations

Throughout the day, a CNA is responsible for the frequent, routine gathering of vital signs, depending on doctors' orders. You can be on a standard four-hour schedule for gathering vitals, or you could be taking them up to every hour or even every 30 minutes in some situations. Daily observations are also a vital component of the role of the CNA.

The following are types of vital signs and observations CNAs are responsible for:

- **Blood Pressure**—This can be both manual and machine-based.
- **Temperature**—This can be completed using an oral thermometer, rectal thermometer, forehead thermometer, or ear canal thermometer, depending on state requirements.
- **Pulse**—This is the number of heartbeats per minute that are counted using the patient's wrist or neck. This may also be collected using a machine-based tool.
- **Respirations**—The number of breaths taken in a minute. This is typically done through observation of the chest cavity rising and falling. Temperature, pulse, and respirations are three common measurements that together make up what is often abbreviated as "TPR" on a patient's chart.
- **Pain Level**—This is typically reported using a scale of 1-10 or sometimes 1-5.
- **Weight**—This can be done on a traditional standing scale. However, some hospital beds can determine weight. In addition, there are roll-on scales for use with wheelchair-using or non-weight bearing residents.

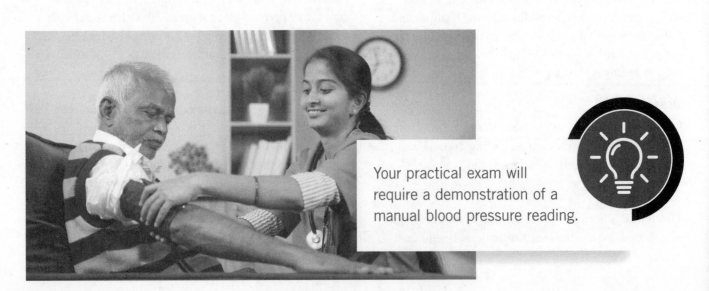

Your practical exam will require a demonstration of a manual blood pressure reading.

- **Oxygen Saturation**—This is completed through a pulse oximeter. Oxygen saturation levels can vary based on patient condition, but normal readings can range from 95%-100%. Individuals with lung conditions, however, can have normal concentrations of 88%-92%. Each patient will have a threshold for acceptable ranges of this, and it is important to correctly document this number quickly, especially if you think the number is too low.

- **The Resident's Five Senses**—Are they reporting any changes in hearing, vision, taste, smell, or touch? This would include numbness, tingling, double vision, etc.

Please see the table below for other daily observations.

Call Lights and Assistance

Although you have assigned tasks for each patient every day, you will also be expected to respond to as-needed requests. A **call light** is a tool provided to every patient for use when they require assistance, and no one is present in their room. In addition, there are emergency buttons in the bathroom or around the patient's neck that they can press if they are experiencing an emergency, such as a fall, tightness in the chest, etc. The emergency button signals a facility-wide alarm and requires any person that is nearby to respond immediately. However, the call light is often monitored by a CNA or office person at a centralized nurses' station or front desk.

Call lights should always be in reach of the patient whether they are sleeping, lack full-body movement, or are cognitively impaired. They need access to call for help at any time of the day or night. In fact, it is illegal to remove a call light from a patient's reach, no matter how frustrating a repeat caller may be. CNAs and HHAs should encourage patients to use call lights for any type of cares, including bathroom needs, positioning, and transferring out of bed. Patients should use call lights for personal needs and wants as well, such as a drink of water, help to reach a book, assistance with finding a TV show, or help with going to an activity. Always offer water and an opportunity to toilet during every call light response. This can help you keep your patient hydrated and avoid repeat trips in the future. Repeated call light usage can be a sign of boredom or anxiety. Try to work through what the patient is trying

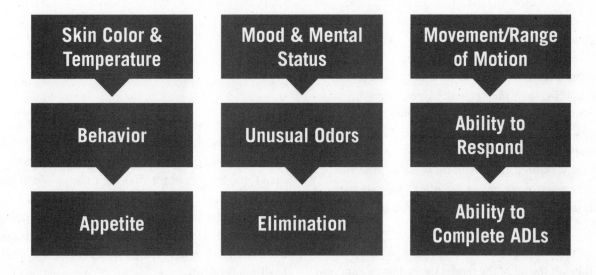

Daily Observations

Skin Color & Temperature	Mood & Mental Status	Movement/Range of Motion
Behavior	Unusual Odors	Ability to Respond
Appetite	Elimination	Ability to Complete ADLs

to communicate. If they are bored, invite them out into the hall, to an activity, or near the nurses' station if no one is available to spend time with them in their room.

Remember that a call light is a patient's only means of communicating their needs aside from yelling (which can be extremely stressful) or getting out of bed unsupervised (impossible for some, dangerous for many). Be respectful whenever you answer the call light.

Meals, Cleaning, and General Upkeep

As a CNA or HHA, you will be expected to transport patients to the cafeteria or dining room and also to assist with delivering their meal. Many patients may not feel up to leaving their rooms, so it is also part of your role to deliver meals to their rooms as needed. You may also be asked to provide some light cleaning and general upkeep of the common areas and rooms. However, there is typically housekeeping staff that is responsible for the bulk of this.

As you get a resident ready for a meal, discuss the menu. Take time to learn the menu in order to communicate what choices are available (if any are available). Begin the process of positively promoting the meal so that your patient is eager and more apt to want to eat upon arrival. Since many residents and patients struggle to eat, it is important to highlight any favorite components of the meal for them. This might be the coffee, juice, meat, or dessert.

When you transport the patient to the dining area, pay attention to who they are friends with and try to seat them by someone they enjoy being near. Also, talk about this person as you are transporting them. Mealtime is often the most social time of the day. You are promoting their mental health by encouraging conversations during meals. Do not ignore nonverbal patients. Just because they cannot talk and may require physical assistance to eat does not mean they do not enjoy conversation. Talk about the world around you, current events, or upcoming activities. Generate the conversation but look for feedback from them via their facial cues as well.

Present meals to bedridden patients in a positive manner. Take off the lid of the food if they allow you and

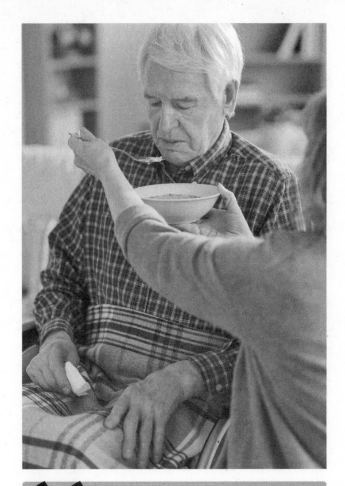

> Mealtime is often the most social time of the day. You are promoting their mental health by encouraging conversations during meals.

set it up, identifying the food as it is arranged. Place the silverware, fill up any water cups, and cut up meat if needed. Your goal is to inspire the patient to eat even though they cannot leave their room. You may also ask if they would like the window open or a TV show turned on. Clean up empty or used meal trays as soon as the resident indicates they are finished. Having a clean and orderly space promotes positive mental health in residents.

MINI-QUIZ: ROLES AND RESPONSIBILITIES

Directions: Read each question below and choose the correct answer from the four choices provided. Only one choice is correct, so choose carefully.

1. Which of the following requires additional certification above and beyond the basic CNA license?

   A. Pericare

   B. Blood glucose monitoring

   C. Assisting with pressure ulcers

   D. Positioning bedridden patients

2. Toileting also includes which type of care?

   A. Dressing

   B. Bathing

   C. Catheter care

   D. Grooming

3. Pericare requires cleanup of which area?

   A. Face

   B. Arms and armpits

   C. Mouth

   D. Genital area

4. The abbreviation TPR refers to what vital signs?

   A. Temperature, Pulse, Respirations

   B. Thermometer, Pulse Oximeter, Respiratory

   C. Temperature, Pulse, Range of Motion

   D. Touch, Plan, Review

5. What does a pulse oximeter read?

   A. Blood pressure

   B. Respirations

   C. Oxygen saturation

   D. Temperature

6. Which of the following is a good oxygen saturation?

   A. 97%

   B. 10%

   C. 50%

   D. 75%

7. A resident may press their call light

   A. outside of mealtimes.

   B. anytime between 7 a.m. and 7 p.m.

   C. after hours only.

   D. 24 hours a day.

8. Which of the following is a daily activity that is the responsibility of a CNA?

   A. Passing medications

   B. Drawing blood

   C. Performing skin ulcer checks

   D. Taking patients to doctors' appointments

9. Pain is usually documented using

   A. a number scale.

   B. medical terminology.

   C. correlating letters.

   D. symbols.

10. Which of the following measures the number of heartbeats per minute?

   A. Temperature

   B. Respirations

   C. Pulse

   D. Oxygen saturation

ANSWER KEY AND EXPLANATIONS

1. B	3. D	5. C	7. D	9. A
2. C	4. A	6. A	8. C	10. C

1. **The correct answer is B.** Blood glucose monitoring requires additional certification. Pericare (choice A), assisting with pressure ulcers (choice C) and positioning bedridden patients (choice D) are all duties allowed with the basic CNA certification.

2. **The correct answer is C.** Although a patient with a catheter does not void into a commode, care of their catheter falls under toileting. Dressing (choice A), bathing (choice B), and grooming (choice D) are all cares but are not related to toileting.

3. **The correct answer is D.** Pericare refers to the genitals and groin area. The face (choice A), arms and armpits (choice B) and mouth (choice C) are not part of pericare.

4. **The correct answer is A.** TPR stands for Temperature, Pulse, and Respirations. The other choices are incorrect.

5. **The correct answer is C.** A pulse oximeter reads oxygen saturation. Some will also include pulse. They are not used for blood pressure (choice A), respirations (choice B), or temperature (choice D).

6. **The correct answer is A.** The highest oxygen saturation is 100%. The closer you are to this number, the better your oxygen saturation is. 75% (choice D), 50% (choice C) and 10% choice B) are all too low and require oxygen assistance.

7. **The correct answer is D.** The call light can be used any time, day or night. It is the lifeline of the patient. There can never be restrictions placed around proper hours that they can use the light; thus, all other answers are incorrect.

8. **The correct answer is C.** Skin ulcer checks can be performed during patient dressing, grooming, toileting, and bathing. Passing medications (choice A) is the responsibility of the nurse. Drawing blood (choice B) can only be delegated to a CNA with an additional certification. Taking patients to doctor's appointments (choice D) usually falls to transportation and a nurse.

9. **The correct answer is A.** Pain is usually documented using a number scale of 1-10, or sometimes 1-5. Medical terminology (choice B) does not apply when documenting, and correlating letters (choice C) and symbols (choice D) are both incorrect.

10. **The correct answer is C.** Pulse is the number of heartbeats per minute. Temperature (choice A) is the degree of heat within your body. Respirations (choice B) are the breaths taken in a minute. Oxygen saturation (choice D) is the amount of oxygen present in your body.

COMMUNICATION

Effective communication is important in medical settings so that the facility, healthcare professionals, and patients understand what is happening and can function properly. Communication is effective only if everyone involved understands what is being shared or said and knows what to do with it. This means that communication should also be bidirectional. Patients should not only understand what you are saying but they also should be able to voice any concerns or questions that they have.

Types of Communication

Communication encompasses all types of interactions between people. It is not only how and what you speak; it is also the way you speak and your body language. In addition, the way information is presented can say just as much as the words and images used. There are four main types of communication: verbal, nonverbal, written, and visual.

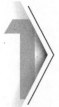

Verbal

Verbal communication includes the words you speak, including word choice and tone. Your **tone** is how you say something and the way you speak to someone else. Pay attention to volume, articulation, and speed. Speaking too loud or too soft can make it difficult for the patient to understand you. Work to speak with a neutral or uplifting tone, even when delivering instructions that may be difficult or upsetting to the patient. Your tone can help steer the conversation. Mumbling or speaking too fast are common problems when speaking with others that are not native speakers. Work to clearly articulate your words and slow down when giving instructions. It can be difficult to try and comply with instructions if they were spoken too quietly, unclearly, or too fast.

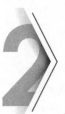

Nonverbal

Nonverbal communication is everything you don't say, including body language, facial expressions, and silences. Close to 90% of our communication is nonverbal. Using **positive body language** signifies to your patient that you are open to communicating with them. Positive body language includes nodding when listening, avoiding crossed arms, and facing the person when they are talking. Pay attention to your body language when speaking with others—it is possible to say positive things but communicate negatively with your body. For example, you might say, "Good morning Mrs. Smith! I'm so happy to see you!" with your words, but if you are crossing your arms, you are actually conveying the opposite emotion.

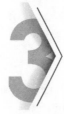

Written

Written communication is anything you write down. Your words in documentation should be clear, correct, and objective. Unless you are asked for your professional opinion about something, everything you document should be clinically accurate without any of your own personal thoughts or emotions included. You can and should include any comments or concerns you may have in the dialogue section of the documentation. Just remember that all medical documentation is a legal document and can be used in a court of law if necessary. When writing, keep the patient and quality care in the forefront of your mind.

Visual

Visual communication relies on images to communicate. It's essential to choose culturally sensitive images whenever you have to use visual communication. In addition, any visuals that you use for menus, ADLs, and activities should be explained to the patient. Do not assume that the patient will automatically understand the visual aids. If you just assume that every visual is brand new, it will help every person you interact with.

Verbal Skills

As discussed, verbal communication needs to be understood by all participants in the conversation. Verbal communication is precisely as it sounds—the act of spoken conversation between two or more individuals. All skills in verbal communication are important, but there are a few that we will highlight for their importance in the medical field.

Feedback

Feedback is a communication technique for providing a patient with specific constructive information. This information is essential for a patient to understand what they need to do in the future with their treatment. This is also helpful to motivate a patient to continue with a new task, such as transferring into and out of a wheelchair. Try to construct your feedback in a positive fashion, even if you are needing the patient to do something different.

Validation

Validation is the process of verifying what a patient has just said to let them know that you understand and are considering what they are saying. This is a very necessary verbal skill as many residents and patients do not feel "heard" by care providers. You do not have to agree with the patient to validate what they are saying.

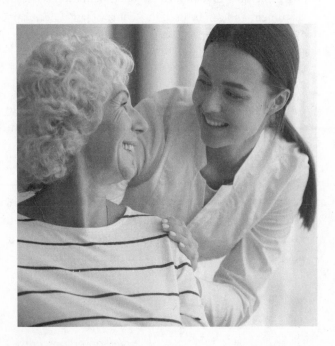

Clarification

Clarification is the process of improving the understanding of a confusing message. This is important because there are many different terms in the medical field and confusion can occur for both patients and medical personnel in different specialties. Don't ever be afraid to ask for clarification. Performing ADLs without complete clarity can be dangerous. In addition, ask for clarification when working with the patient. You and the patient are, in essence, a team—both of you need to understand what the other needs to effectively and safely provide care.

Summary

Summary is used to emphasize the main ideas or feelings that were discussed in a conversation. Accurate summary helps to highlight important ideas for all parties involved. This can be a terrific tool to ensure the patient understands what is being requested of them. In addition, the care provider can summarize processes so there is no confusion moving forward.

Nonverbal Skills

Nonverbal skills can be just as important as verbal skills at times. Nonverbal skills include conversation features like demeanor, tone, and active listening. If nonverbal skills are not used effectively during communication, then the other parties may consider you to be indifferent or rude and may refuse to listen. These are the main components to pay attention to when focusing on nonverbal communication.

Active Listening

Active listening is the most important nonverbal communication skill to possess because it allows you to take in information and validate the speaker. To show you are listening, face the speaker, make eye contact (if culturally appropriate), and nod your head. While the patient is speaking, make sure you are giving them your full attention and listening to the entire message they are conveying instead of listening to respond. When they are finished speaking, repeat their ideas back to them to show that you've listened and understand. Validating a patient's ideas will help them feel encouraged to continue sharing their ideas with you. Many patients complain that care providers do not truly listen when they are speaking. By being an active listener, you can ensure that you do not fall into this category.

Demeanor

Demeanor is how someone carries themselves, also called body language. Your posture, the placement of your arms (crossed or open), and whether you face someone when they speak are all part of your demeanor. Having a poor demeanor, such as indifference towards a serious topic, will tell the other person that you are not concerned with the conversation and are not listening to what is being communicated. Patients should always feel that you are invested in what they are saying as they are the reason you come to work every day.

Facial Expression

This technically falls under demeanor and should also be taken into consideration when acting professionally. This area can be difficult for some people as we have little control over our resting face or how we look when we are thinking. That being said, make an effort to emit positive facial expressions when in the presence of a patient. They should always feel that you want to be around them, not that they are a burden or a chore.

Appearance

This is extremely important when working in a professional setting. Having a professional appearance will help the individuals you are communicating with know that you are a professional and are serious about your work.

CONFIDENTIALITY
All patient information is protected by confidentiality laws to provide a safe and private space for the patient to receive care. Several terms are important to understand when ensuring confidentiality is upheld during all communication related to the patient.

TERM	DEFINITION
Informed Consent	when a patient is informed of treatment and medical care, understands the risks and benefits, and agrees to the plan. This can also apply to other areas of life, such as financial consent.
Release of Information	a signed form that allows you to release information to others outside of your immediate care team. It is important to honor and respect your patient's decisions. If this is not signed and specified for outside providers, you cannot legally provide any personal information about your patient.
Privacy	includes both privacy about their medical care and privacy while receiving care. For example, shutting the curtain when the resident is undressing.
Indiscretion	an accidental sharing of confidential information. It is not done on purpose, but it can unintentionally harm the patient. Avoid talking about patients outside of your care team. Also, ensure your conversation about patients is centered on care and not on gossip. All patients can be difficult at times, but there is a difference between asking for support and criticizing patients.
Breach of Confidentiality	an intentional sharing of private, sensitive information outside of the care team. Some family members may try to get you to share information that the patient has not released to them. It is your duty as a care provider to never release sensitive medical information unless the proper forms are in place and signed.
HIPAA	stands for Health Insurance Portability and Accountability Act. This was created by the government in 1996 and protects the patient's privacy as it is transmitted between providers, health insurance companies, and other agencies (such as auto insurance companies and the patient's workplace). The goal of HIPAA is to protect the patient's privacy while also ensuring the flow of transmission is effective and efficient.

MINI-QUIZ: COMMUNICATION

Directions: Read each question below and choose the correct answer from the four choices provided. Only one choice is correct, so choose carefully.

1. An example of closed nonverbal communication is

   A. nodding your head.

   B. looking down.

   C. crossing your arms.

   D. remaining silent.

2. How someone carries themselves, including their body language, is also called

   A. validation.

   B. feedback.

   C. demeanor.

   D. indiscretion.

3. Which of the following would work best when needing further explanation on an assigned duty?

   A. Feedback

   B. Validation

   C. Summary

   D. Clarification

4. Which of the following is NOT one of the main four types of communication?

   A. Comprehensive

   B. Visual

   C. Nonverbal

   D. Written

5. Which of the following may or may not be a sign of active listening depending on culture?

   A. Nodding

   B. Open body language

   C. Eye contact

   D. Positive facial expression

6. When communicating, using physical gestures can help those with _____ deficits.

   A. hearing

   B. memory

   C. visual

   D. hearing or memory

7. A resident is observed with their head down and eyes closed throughout the entire morning care routine. They are still able to communicate verbally, but they are only answering basic questions. Which of the following may be true?

   A. They are not ready to wake up.

   B. They are relaxed and enjoying their care.

   C. They are excited and ready for the day.

   D. They are thinking about the rest of their day.

8. A nonverbal resident repeatedly tightens their face whenever green vegetables are presented. What might they be trying to communicate?

   A. They are eager to eat.

   B. They are struggling to chew.

   C. They do not like this type of food.

   D. They are enjoying the food.

9. A memory care resident moans frequently during Hoyer lift transfers, but their face does not display any tension. What might they be trying to communicate?

   A. They are scared.

   B. They are angry.

   C. They are excited.

   D. They are tired.

10. A resident signs a form without the nurse properly explaining what they are signing. What healthcare process or procedure was not followed?

    A. Informed consent

    B. HIPAA rights

    C. Confidentiality

    D. Privacy

NOTES

ANSWER KEY AND EXPLANATIONS

1. C	3. D	5. C	7. A	9. C
2. C	4. A	6. D	8. C	10. A

1. **The correct answer is C.** Crossing your arms is an example of closed nonverbal communication as it closes your body off from receiving information. Nodding your head (choice A) is a type of open communication. Looking down (choice B) and remaining silent (choice D) can be perceived as negative cues but are highly dependent on culture.

2. **The correct answer is C.** Demeanor is another term for body language. Validation (choice A) and feedback (choice B) are both types of verbal communication. Indiscretion (choice D) is an accidental breach of confidentiality.

3. **The correct answer is D.** Clarification is the process by which you request further explanation after hearing instructions. Feedback (choice A) is the process of providing information after receiving information. Validation (choice B) is the process of ensuring that the other person's message is heard and not just through casual listening. Summary (choice C) is when you recap the conversation in a short and concise format.

4. **The correct answer is A.** Comprehensive communication is not an official type of communication. Visual (choice B), nonverbal (choice C), and written (choice D) are three out of the four types, with verbal being the fourth.

5. **The correct answer is C.** Eye contact can be a sign of active listening, but the use of it is culturally specific. Nodding (choice A), open body language (choice B), and positive facial expressions are all associated with active listening.

6. **The correct answer is D.** Both hearing impaired and intellectually compromised individuals can benefit from physical gestures in combination with spoken word. Choices A, B, and C are incorrect.

7. **The correct answer is A.** When someone has their eyes closed and head down, they are not open in their body language. Couple that with the timing of the care (early morning), and it is most likely that they are not ready to wake up. The other options are all positive and would involve some type of open body language.

8. **The correct answer is C.** When a person is nonverbal, their facial cues are extremely important. A tightened face demonstrates tension, which, in this case, is only occurring when a certain type of food is presented. It is important for the CNA/HHA to pay attention to nonverbal communication, especially when verbal communication is not an option. All other choices are incorrect.

9. **The correct answer is C.** Moaning without tension can often be an expression of excitement among those with cognitive deficits. Make sure to verbally articulate what you think they are feeling and check for understanding. Do they provide eye contact or a smile or nod when you label it as excitement? Do they seem eager to enter the lift? All of these are positive signs. If they were scared (choice A) or angry (choice B), they would have tension in their face. If they were tired (choice D), there would be other nonverbal cues present, such as slouching.

10. **The correct answer is A.** Whenever a patient is asked to sign something, they must be provided an appropriate explanation of what the document is and how it will be used. The nurse did not do this; thus, the patient could not provide informed consent. HIPAA rights (choice B) are not received by signing papers but are afforded to all patients. Confidentiality (choice C) and privacy (choice D) may have been provided, but the question does not state how the form was presented (in a hallway, in a private room, etc.).

RESIDENT RIGHTS AND LEGAL ISSUES

All patients, regardless of their health status, have client rights that ensure both ethical and legal treatment. There are laws in place in the US to ensure the safe and ethical treatment of patients. In addition, there are rules and guidelines within a facility to protect every resident. In this section, we will cover the rights of long-term care (LTC) residents. They are often the most compromised and the most isolated, as their condition is chronic and often terminal.

We will cover the following topics:

- Resident Rights
- Legal Documents and Decision Making
- The Long-Term Care Ombudsman (LTCO)
- Adult Protective Services (APS)
- State Licensing Agency and Surveys

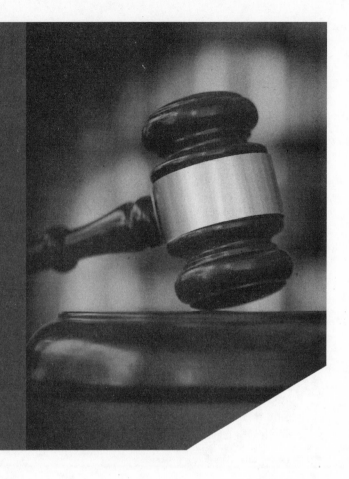

Resident Rights

Every long-term care (LTC) resident has basic rights referred to as their **Resident Rights** or the **Patient Bill of Rights**. Every LTC facility must have the rights posted in an easily visible place, must provide new residents with a copy in their preferred language, and must provide updated copies annually or whenever a resident has a new care plan in place.

The following is a list of the basic resident rights for every resident:

1. **The right to information in a preferred language.**
   Information should always be presented in the resident's preferred written language. Never assume this is the same language you speak with them.

2. **The right to independent choices based on needs and wants.**
   Regardless of medical limitations, every resident should be consulted when making decisions that affect them.

3. **The right to participate in all aspects of care.**
   Every meeting regarding a patient's care should include a personal invite to the patient/resident, even if they typically turn it down. In addition, they should also be consulted about who they want to attend the meeting, like family members, friends, etc. Just because the patient or resident's child or other loved one wants to be at the meeting doesn't mean they can be there. Unless there is a legal document on file requiring that a particular person be at such a meeting (if there's a guardianship in place, etc.), no family member or friend must be there, even if it makes it easier for the facility.

4. **The right to privacy and confidentiality.**
Every patient is granted basic confidentiality through HIPAA privacy rules among providers. It is not your place to inform or update family members or friends about a patient's medical treatment without the expressed consent of the resident. In addition, all ADLs should be done with the utmost privacy, even if the resident doesn't appear to notice. What they can communicate and how they feel may be different. Assume they prefer extreme privacy unless otherwise communicated by the resident. Residents are also granted privacy rights regarding access to communication with others outside of the facility. Access to a private phone is required for all residents. Staff may not monitor calls or limit them without a medical or legal reason.

5. **The right to participate in preferred community-based interests including social and religious activities.**
There is a common assumption that a resident must get permission to leave the facility. However, this is not true. They simply need to notify the staff properly so their whereabouts are known. The resident is still a member of the community and should never feel that they cannot leave if they have the means to do so.

6. **The right to complain without fear of repercussions.**
There is an internal complaint policy in every LTC facility. In addition, the Long-Term Care Ombudsman monitors every facility and is there to assist a resident if they have a complaint they cannot, or are afraid to, resolve with the staff alone.

7. **The right to be treated without discrimination, abuse, neglect, and restraints.**
Instances of patient abuse and neglect do occur, even in facilities with hundreds of residents and dozens of workers. It is up to you as their care provider to ensure that you treat them with respect and dignity and report any suspicious behavior, bruising, etc.

8. **The right to visits from anyone the patient chooses.**
Unless a family member has guardianship, they cannot and should not restrict any visitors. This is true even if they have power of attorney (POA). POA does not remove the free will of the resident. A patient is allowed visits from anyone of their choosing, and staff should help to schedule visits if the resident requests assistance. In addition, it is a breach of privacy to report visits to family or friends without guardianship.

9. **The right to adequate medical care.**
This should be for all residents, regardless of payor source.

10. **The right to organize and participate in a resident-centered council.**
Every facility is required by law to have a resident-run council. Their role is to be the voice of the residents within the facility, discussing important topics, such as common complaints, menus, activities, and anything of their choosing. Part of this meeting can be completely closed, without any facility staff present if desired.

11. **The right to proper notification and participation in the transfer and discharge process.**
A resident cannot be transferred or discharged without proper notification and with a safe and realistic plan in place. A social worker at the facility must create a full discharge or transfer plan for all their medical needs.

4

Legal Documents and Decision-making

Many residents in a LTC facility have some type of legal documents on file for decision-making related to financial and medical choices. However, there are often misconceptions about what each document allows and what it doesn't allow. We will review the three types of legal documents you may encounter and the permissions and restrictions of each.

TYPES OF LEGAL DOCUMENTS			
	POWER OF ATTORNEY (POA)	**CONSERVATORSHIP**	**GUARDIANSHIP**
Appointment	• Not appointed by a court of law. • Can be revoked by the resident at any time.	• Appointed by a court of law. • Legally binding and must request removal officially.	• Appointed by a court of law. • Legally binding and must request removal officially.
Decision-Making	• Common for financial or medical decisions. • Resident retains their own decision-making rights.	• Usually only used for financial management. • Resident's finances are handled by conservator, but all other decisions are made by the resident.	• Applies to all decisions that affect the resident. • Every aspect of care is handled by the guardian. The guardian is responsible for all decisions.
Overrides	POA cannot override any decisions made by the resident.	Conservator can override financial decisions only.	The guardian can override ALL decisions made by the resident.
Resident's Wants	POA can act in place of the resident only when the resident requests or when they are incapacitated (coma, stroke, etc.).	Conservator can make lateral decisions about finances only, regardless of the resident's wants, although their wants should be considered.	Guardian can make lateral decisions about all care, although the resident's wants should be considered if possible.
Meetings	POAs do not need to be present at every meeting but can be at the request of the resident.	Must be present at any meeting that has to do with finances only. They should not be invited to meetings beyond their scope.	Must be present at all meetings related to the resident, regardless of topic.

The Long-Term Care Ombudsman (LTCO)

All 50 states plus Washington D.C. and Puerto Rico have a full-time state-appointed Long-Term Care Ombudsman (LTCO) who ensures that residents of all LTC facilities receive proper and adequate care. A state can have a team of county-level ombudsman that assist them in advocating for residents, depending on the size and funding of the state. The role of the LTCO is unique and unlike any other.

The following list provides important components of the role of this patient-centered advocate.

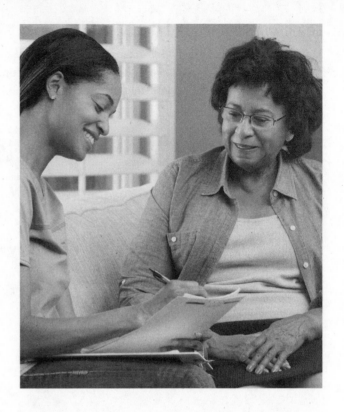

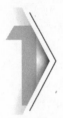

The LTCO advocates for the patient's wants and needs from the patient's perspective. The goal of the LTCO is to ensure the wants and needs of the resident are met. It is up to the care team to figure out how those wants and needs can be executed in a safe manner. Sometimes, the patient's wants may go against sound medical treatments, preferred scheduling for the facility, and the voice of the family members. One example of this is a patient with lung cancer who wants to smoke. The LTCO will work with the patient to advocate for their decision, even though it is obviously unhealthy. The care team must figure out how to honor the patient's want by, for example, leaving the oxygen tank inside the building while the resident smokes outside.

The LTCO's documentation and notes about a patient are confidential, even in legal matters. Unlike doctors, therapists, and other professionals, the documentation that an LTCO must keep regarding an LTC resident cannot be subpoenaed through a court of law. These records are protected through the ombudsman program and LTCO have immunity regarding testifying about their conversations with the resident in question.

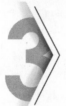

The LTCO works together with Adult Protection Services, law enforcement, and the state licensing agency to ensure residents receive proper care and treatment. If a resident asks for help with a situation that includes abuse or neglect, the LTCO will involve all legal entities necessary at the resident's direction. Remember, the LTCO works for the resident and no one else—not the family, the facility, or the government.

Staff can anonymously report concerns regarding resident rights to the LTCO. A nurse's aide is a patient's closest care provider, seeing the resident every day and hearing their concerns. If you observe anything that causes you concern, you can report it to the LTCO. If the resident expresses a desire to work through their grievance, you can direct them to the LTCO number that must be obviously posted in a visible and easily accessible location. Any information you provide to the LTCO will never be disclosed to your facility if you request anonymity.

Adult Protective Services (APS)

The **Adult Protective Services (APS)** program is run at the county level in every county nationwide. Their role is to ensure the safety, independence, and quality of life for at-risk adults. "At-risk" is defined as an adult that is over 18 and susceptible to abuse, neglect, and mistreatment. This can include those with intellectual and mental disabilities, gravely ill patients, and geriatric individuals. APS investigates allegations of abuse, neglect, and mistreatment of at-risk and elderly adults, both in the community and in LTC facilities. APS also addresses emergent, basic needs, including food, water, and shelter. If needed, APS will involve law enforcement to ensure a safe environment for the adult in question.

At-risk adults have the right to refuse help or refuse to speak to APS. If there is grave danger without their intervention, APS members may petition the courts for emergency guardianship to ensure that the adult receives lifesaving medical or mental health treatment.

Each state has laws around **mandated reporters** for at-risk adults. These are professionals who are required to report cases of suspected abuse or neglect to appropriate agencies. Medical professionals like CNAs and HHAs often fall under this category. When making a report, APS will ask for as much information as possible about the person, the suspected mistreatment, and how to contact this person. They will also ask for your personal information if you are inclined to give it. In most cases, mandated reporters do not remain anonymous as they may be called in to testify under a court of law. If you decide to remain anonymous, it can be extremely difficult for members of APS to fully investigate the case. Laws exist that protect mandated reporters from retaliation, so you will be safe if you ever report suspected abuse or neglect.

Common Types of Abuse and Neglect

Financial Exploitation: Misappropriation of funds by the POA, an in-home care provider, or a live-in trusted friend.	**Physical Abuse:** Includes beating, scratching, biting, and bruising. Can sometimes be detected as strange bruises or varying degrees of patient wounds that are healing.	**Verbal Abuse:** Includes yelling, cursing, racial and sexual slurs, and any other words that seek to demean, control, or belittle the adult.	**Emotional/ Psychological Abuse:** Can be difficult to prove at times as abusers in this category are excellent manipulators. They often convince the victim they are bad or a burden on the abuser.
Sexual Abuse: Includes rape, molestation, grooming, and taking sexual advantage of a geriatric or cognitively impaired adult. If they cannot give informed consent, it is not consensual.	**Medical Neglect:** The denial of required medical care, including access to necessary medication, such as insulin, pain medications, and home-health services.	**Imprisonment:** The unlawful entrapment of an at-risk adult against their will. This is often discovered when a patient is not coming to their scheduled appointments.	**Abandonment:** The willful deserting of an at-risk adult who is under your care without ensuring there is a plan and another person in place to care for them.

State Licensing Agency and Surveys

Every long-term care facility is licensed at the state level. Different agencies are responsible for this in each state, but the rules and regulations remain the same. Every LTC facility is surveyed yearly to ensure that they are complying with federal standards and conditions. Just like a restaurant is inspected, rated, and sometimes given a list of infractions, regulatory agencies can inspect and report on nursing homes as well. The LTC facility is given a list of its deficiencies, and it has 30 days to make the corrections to renew its license.

Surveys include interviews with all levels of staff, including CNAs and HHAs. Be open and honest about your experience, the care provided to the residents, and any concerns you may have. Your grievances during a survey are not documented specifically, but rather compiled in one large report. Surveyors can and do come out if someone files a license-specific complaint that involves the federal regulations for LTC facilities. These types of urgent investigations are similar in fashion to APS, but it is an organization that is under investigation rather than a person. If your workplace is ever investigated in this manner, simply be upfront and honest about how it is run, what you are asked to do, and the type of care you can provide to your residents.

Surveyors work closely with the LTCO and look to them to give an overview of how the facility has operated throughout the year, any concerns they have as the county-level oversight provider, and what they would like to see changed or investigated. Deficiencies are rated on a level of severity. If a facility receives deficiencies in critical care, such as safety, abuse, or medication management, it can be closed immediately, and all the residents will be moved until it is safe again.

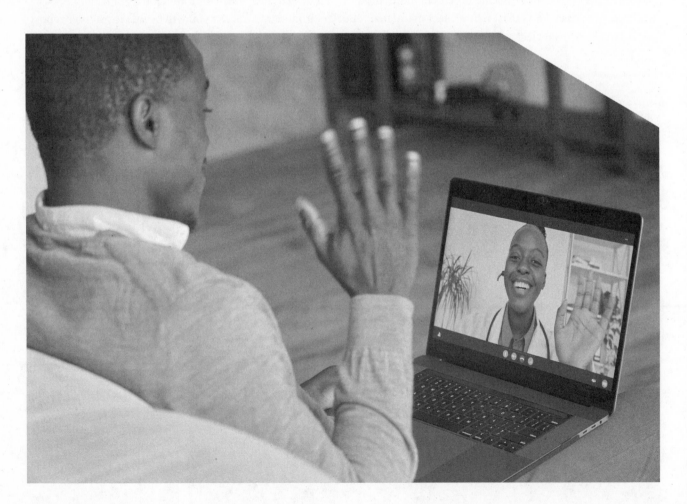

MINI-QUIZ: RESIDENT RIGHTS AND LEGAL ISSUES

Directions: Read each question below and choose the correct answer from the four choices provided. Only one choice is correct, so choose carefully.

1. The legal document that allows for a person to override financial decisions ONLY is called a

   A. power of attorney.

   B. conservatorship.

   C. guardianship.

   D. living will.

2. The person or body that investigates suspected abuse of at-risk adults is called

   A. the Long-Term Care Ombudsman.

   B. Adult Protective Services.

   C. the state ombudsman.

   D. the surveyor.

3. If a resident has dramatically lost weight and is never brought out of her room for meals, she may be experiencing

   A. neglect.

   B. psychological abuse.

   C. financial exploitation.

   D. physical abuse.

4. The right to telephone calls falls under which resident right?

   A. The right to community access

   B. The right to proper and adequate care

   C. The right to privacy

   D. The right to make decisions in care

5. Who can make reports to the Long-Term Care Ombudsman about resident rights issues?

   A. The resident

   B. The staff

   C. A family member

   D. All of the above

6. How often do long-term care facilities have regularly scheduled licensing surveys?

   A. Annually

   B. Every two years

   C. Every six months

   D. As often as needed

7. The licensing regulations that all long-term care facilities must adhere to are approved at the

   A. city level.

   B. county level.

   C. state level.

   D. federal level.

8. An 85-year-old woman who uses a wheelchair just had her nephew move in with her. Neighbors haven't seen the woman leave the house in weeks. They call APS to check in on her. Upon arrival, the worker notices that the kitchen cupboards are bare and the woman's clothes are tattered. During the worker's investigation, she meets the nephew who appears to be well-dressed and of good health. What type of abuse may be occurring?

   A. Sexual abuse

   B. Physical abuse

   C. Financial exploitation

   D. Medical neglect

9. A resident wants to eat ice cream every day for breakfast. The person with Power of Attorney for the resident has forbidden it, and the dietary department is refusing to provide the requested ice cream. The Long-Term Care Ombudsman is advocating for the daily ice cream. What should the facility do?

A. Ask the POA for more information on why they won't allow the ice cream.

B. Set up a meeting with the POA, the dietary department, and the resident to explain why it isn't healthy to eat ice cream for breakfast.

C. Try to convince the POA to change their mind.

D. Listen to the resident and provide ice cream.

10. A resident council must be attended by the

A. facility administrator.

B. Long-Term Care Ombudsman.

C. activities director.

D. residents.

NOTES

ANSWER KEY AND EXPLANATIONS

1. B	**3.** A	**5.** D	**7.** D	**9.** D
2. B	**4.** C	**6.** A	**8.** C	**10.** D

1. **The correct answer is B.** A conservatorship focuses on financial control only. A power of attorney (choice A) does allow for overriding any decisions. A guardianship (choice C) can override all decisions. A living will (choice D) does not relate to decision-making beyond directives for healthcare.

2. **The correct answer is B.** Adult protective services is responsible for investigating suspected abuse against at-risk adults. The Long-Term Care Ombudsman (choice A) is a resident advocate and may work alongside APS. The state ombudsman (choice C) supervises the entire state program. The surveyor (choice D) investigates complaints related to regulatory compliance.

3. **The correct answer is A.** Weight loss is a huge indicator of neglect in a facility. That, coupled with her not being brought out for her meals, is troubling. However, in the case above, there are no other signs of psychological abuse (choice B), financial exploitation (choice C), or physical abuse (choice D), although it is possible and even likely that these may be occurring alongside this neglect.

4. **The correct answer is C.** The right to telephone calls falls under privacy and confidentiality. The other choices are all incorrect in this instance.

5. **The correct answer is D.** Although the Long-Term Care Ombudsman is the voice of the resident, anyone who is concerned about an issue with the resident's rights can and should contact the LTCO for assistance.

6. **The correct answer is A.** Regularly scheduled licensing surveys always occur annually and not every two years (choice B) or every six months (choice C). Complaint-driven surveys can occur as often as needed (choice D).

7. **The correct answer is D.** All LTC facilities must adhere to licensing regulations that are approved at the federal level. Depending on the state (choice C), county (choice B), and city (choice A), there may be additional levels of regulations required.

8. **The correct answer is C.** The fact that the nephew's condition appears in such contrast to the woman's could be a red flag pointing to financial exploitation, especially as no food seems to be present in the house. There is no evidence of sexual abuse (choice A), physical abuse (choice B), or medical neglect (choice D) based on the information provided.

9. **The correct answer is D.** The POA has no legal recourse regarding decision-making for the resident. If the resident wants ice cream and does not have a guardianship in place, their wishes should be honored, not the wishes of the POA (choices A, B, and C).

10. **The correct answer is D.** The residents are the only required participants in a resident-run council. They can invite the administrator (choice A), the Long-Term Care Ombudsman (choice B), and the activities director (choice C) if desired, but it is not required. They can request that their meeting be completely closed from staff and outsiders.

SUMMING IT UP

- The bulk of your work as a CNA or HHA encompasses Activities of Daily Living (ADLs) including feeding, bathing, dressing, grooming, toileting, and other activities.

- A CNA is often asked to gather, prepare, and sanitize necessary equipment for the nurse to use.

- Throughout the day, a CNA is responsible for the routine gathering of vital signs, including blood pressure, temperature, pulse, respirations, pain level, weight, oxygen saturation, and the patient's five senses.

- A call light is a tool provided to every patient for use when they require assistance and no one is present in their room. In addition, there are emergency buttons in the bathroom or around the patient's neck that they can press if they are experiencing an emergency.

  o Call lights should always be in reach of the patient.

- As a CNA or HHA, you will be expected to transport patients to the cafeteria, deliver meals, and provide light cleaning and general upkeep of common areas.

- Effective communication is important in medical settings so that the facility, healthcare professionals, and patients understand what is happening and can function properly.

- Communication encompasses all types of interactions between people, including verbal, nonverbal, written, and visual communication.

  o The most important verbal skills for a CNA or HHA to possess are feedback, validation, clarification, and summary.

  o Nonverbal skills include conversation features like active listening, demeanor, facial expression, and appearance.

- All patient information is protected by confidentiality laws to provide a safe and private space for the patient to receive care.

  o Important ideas to understand regarding patient confidentiality are informed consent, release of information, privacy, indiscretion, breach of confidentiality, and HIPAA.

- There are laws in place in the US to ensure the safe and ethical treatment of patients.

- Every long-term care (LTC) resident has basic rights referred to as their Resident Rights or the Patient Bill of Rights.

- Many residents in a LTC facility have some type of legal documents on file for decision-making related to financial and medical choices. Important ones to know are power of attorney (POA), conservatorship, and guardianship.

- The Long-Term Care Ombudsman (LTCO) is a state-appointed official who ensures that residents of all LTC facilities receive proper and adequate care.

- Adult Protective Services (APS) ensures the safety, independence, and quality of life for at-risk adults by investigating allegations of abuse, neglect, and mistreatment of elderly adults in LTC facilities.

  o Abuse and neglect may include financial exploitation, physical abuse, verbal abuse, emotional/psychological abuse, medical neglect, imprisonment, and abandonment.

- Every LTC facility is surveyed yearly to ensure that it is complying with federal standards and conditions. Surveys include interviews with all levels of staff, including CNAs and HHAs.

ACTIVITIES OF DAILY LIVING (ADLs

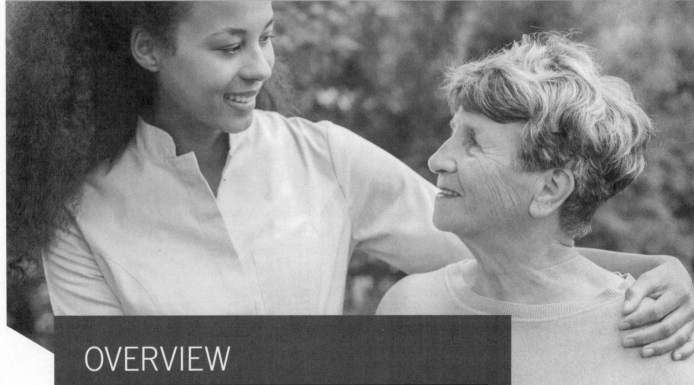

OVERVIEW

»

What are Activities of Daily Living (ADLs)?

Activities of Daily Living (ADLs) are the daily physical needs that people have that are necessary for a healthy state of living and include tasks like eating, drinking, bathing, dressing, or moving around. When discussing ADLs, we will refer to the primary and common ADLs that healthcare professionals frequently perform in a facility setting. They include the following:

1 **Ambulating**—moving from one point to another; walking with or without the use of any ambulatory aids, such as canes or walkers.

2 **Dressing**—dressing oneself; doing so with clothing appropriate for the weather or the occasion.

3 **Personal hygiene**—cleaning and grooming oneself, including bathing, nail care, hair care, and dental care.

4 **Feeding**—physically feeding oneself and, at times, being able to choose a healthy meal.

5 **Continence**—controlling one's bladder and bowels; using a catheter if needed.

6 **Toileting**—navigating to or away from the toilet, using it correctly, and cleaning oneself properly after.

7 **Bathing**—cleaning oneself using a shower, shower chair, or bathtub; includes dressing and undressing, transferring in and out of the shower/chair/tub, and physically and cognitively being able to clean oneself effectively.

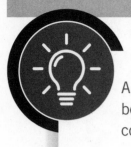

A resident must physically AND cognitively complete an ADL for them to be considered independent. Many residents are physically restricted but are cognitively aware. Remember this when providing care.

When assisting with ADLs, a CNA or HHA should always prioritize the patient's safety and dignity. To keep patients safe, CNAs or HHAs should pay attention to factors like preventing accidents, providing physical support of a patient's body, and honoring dietary restrictions. Preserving a patient's dignity is an important part of ADLs because a CNA or HHA assists a patient with tasks that they may have once been able to do on their own. Keeping care private, engaging the patient in conversation during care, and asking the patient to make decisions about their care preferences can ensure their dignity remains intact.

Issues with mobility, memory, or other factors may cause patients to need assistance with ADLs. Some patients may be able to complete ADLs on their own under a CNA's or HHA's observation and assistance. Other patients may require partial help, meaning that they can complete most or some of the tasks with an aide's assistance. Some patients will require complete care. These patients can no longer perform these daily activities on their own and need full assistance from a CNA or HHA. No matter the level of need, CNAs and HHAs should remember that assisting with ADLs is one of the most important functions of their role.

Assessment for ADLs

Assessing ADLs is an essential process throughout a shift. In the beginning, a patient is generally assessed overall for any assistance needs regarding ADLs. The most common assessment used is the **Katz Index of Independence in Activities of Daily Living**, also referred to as the **Katz Index**.

Katz Index

The Katz Index is a questionnaire checklist used to determine if a patient can or cannot independently perform basic ADLs. The range and number system may differ by facility, but the categories are as follows:

KATZ INDEX		
NUMBER	**LEVEL OF ASSISTANCE**	**DEFINITION**
0	Independent	Resident does not require help of any kind (including verbal cues).
1	Limited Supervision	Resident requires encouragement or cues.
2	Limited Assistance	Resident is highly involved and needs some physical assistance.
3	Extensive Assistance	Resident requires weight-bearing assistance, transfer help, and/or full staff support during part but not all of the activity.

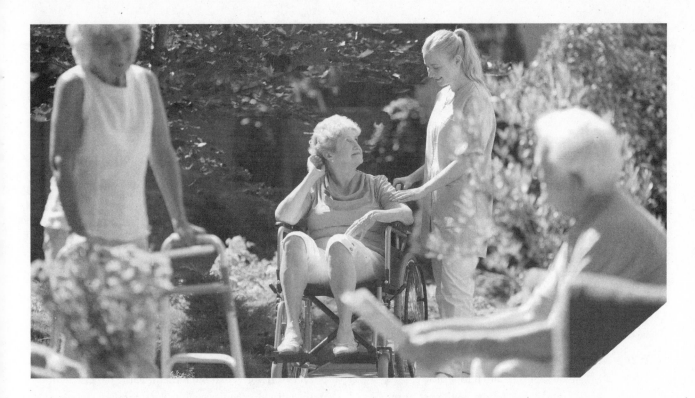

A strong point of the Katz Index is that it helps create a common language between the staff and the patient for their needs. However, if retaken during or after rehabilitation, the Katz Index does not always account for small changes with the patient's abilities. It is important for the CNA or HHA to notice these small changes since they don't always register on the Katz Index.

Assessment is critical in the middle and end of a patient's care, not just the beginning. It should be recognized whenever a patient gains or loses the ability to perform an ADL. Continued assessment helps the CNA notice these changes and helps the patient receive whatever aid they need. CNAs and HHAs document the level of assistance needed each day with basic ADLs to help nurses and doctors create ongoing changes to care plans and treatment.

Promoting Safety and Dignity

Once a CNA or HHA is clear about the patient's level of need and ability regarding ADLs, it is important to determine the best ways to care for that patient, according to their care plan and to their preferences. When making decisions with and for the patient about care, a CNA and HHA should always keep **safety** and

dignity at the forefront of ADL plans and procedures. Sometimes, patients can become embarrassed or upset because of their inability to perform basic ADLs. Leading the way with compassion and know-how will help a CNA or HHA provide the necessary care in a safe and dignified way.

Safety

With all things medical, **safety** should always be a top priority for patients and staff, even in the smallest of tasks. Following some basic procedures and paying attention to a patient's care plan and preferences can help keep them safe. For example, a patient might be allergic to a certain product used in everyday tasks. The CNA or HHA should know which products that patient can and cannot use to avoid allergic reactions. Sometimes, patients may require additional care after a task beyond the standard procedure. Treating each patient as an individual with specific needs can help prevent accidents and keep each patient safe.

In Chapter 6, we will go into more depth about how to keep patients safe, but, for now, the following table provides general safety considerations when caring for a patient who needs assistance with ADLs.

SAFETY CONSIDERATIONS

TOPIC	ACTION	EXAMPLE
Accidents	Assistance should be summoned immediately if there is an accident or safety hazard of any kind.	• If a patient has an accident that could be embarrassing, such as falling while trying to make it to the bathroom, do not yell out or notify multiple people. • Use the bedside call for a nurse and stay with the patient.
Body Movements	Be sure to follow proper movement and support procedures when aiding a patient.	• Do not move a patient in a manner that is not a part of the procedure. • Supporting the patient should also precisely follow the given procedures. Failure to do so can result in a patient falling or getting injured.
Liquids	When serving a patient liquid to eat or drink, make sure to pay attention to temperature and fill level.	• Never fill a mug or bowl with a hot liquid to the top. • There should be space between the top of the liquid and the top of the container to prevent spilling.
Eating	Make sure food and drinks are at an appropriate temperature, size, and consistency for the patient to consume.	• If the temperature is too cold, it can shock a patient, and if it is too hot, it can burn them. Some patients will struggle with larger pieces of food, and if they struggle enough with swallowing or chewing, they will be put on a mechanical soft diet with ground and puréed food.
Bathing	When bathing a patient, make sure to clean their body in an order that will prevent infection and be sure to check water temperature.	• Wash a patient's perineal area last to minimize the spread of bacteria. Use a towel or sponge for one area, then use a new and clean one when moving on to a new area. • Ensure the bathing water is at a good temperature, reheating or cooling as necessary throughout the bath.
Cutting Toenails	Know what tasks a CNA or HHA is responsible for completing. There are some simple tasks that should only be done by a nurse or doctor, like cutting toenails.	• A nurse or doctor almost always cuts toenails. Toenails need to be cut straight across to prevent damage to the skin and ingrown toenails.

Dignity

Helping a patient to feel comfortable while assisting with an ADL helps to preserve their **dignity**, especially if they are being helped for the first time or have recently started needing help with a new task. Dignity is the patient's self-pride or self-respect, and helping to preserve it shows them that they are worthy of respect and that their life has value. Loss of dignity can affect the patient's emotional state, sometimes causing them to react in anger or causing them to withdraw. CNAs and HHAs can preserve a patient's dignity by having open communication with the patient about their care, being discreet when the patient struggles or has accidents, and having a comprehensive understanding of the patient's needs as outlined in their care plan. It is up to the CNA or HHA to take steps to preserve the patient's dignity while also ensuring that they are physically comfortable.

5

Here are a few ways to help preserve the dignity of a patient during a task:

TIPS TO PRESERVE DIGNITY		
TOPIC	**ACTION**	**EXAMPLE**
Communication	Have a natural conversation with your patient to let them know they are valued and respected. Ask for their input so they know their opinions matter.	• When beginning a new task, talk to the patient in a calm and conversational tone and explain the process. • Ask the patient for input about small decisions like what shoes they want to wear or how they want their hair styled. • Always speak directly to the patient instead of talking about them.
Patient Preferences	Always respect your patient's preferences with the products you use to care for them. You should also allow them to help you with the task if they prefer to and are able.	• Use familiar products like soaps, lotions, or towels. • Dress them in clothing they enjoy or request as long as the clothing is appropriate for the weather and occasion. • If a patient can lift food to their mouth, cut the food for them and then let the resident lift it to their mouth.
Family Input	Talk to the patient's family to get a better understanding of the patient's preferences and personality. Understanding what is important to the patient can help a CNA or HHA better care for and respect the patient.	• Family members may be able to tell you how the patient likes their makeup applied or their hair done. • Family can also identify the patient's spiritual or cultural needs, like wearing a religious headdress or garb. • Always verify this information with the patient if you can before proceeding.
Care Plan	Read the patient's care plan, which thoroughly outlines all the patient's needs and how to perform them.	• Each patient is different, with varying needs and expectations. • Learning about their diagnosis, the actions a CNA or HHA can assist with to care for them, and the desired outcomes of their treatment should be of utmost importance.
Discretion	Be discreet when completing personal care and reporting accidents. Do not openly discuss a patient's private personal care or any accidents.	• When sponge bathing a patient, uncover only what must be cleaned, and cover the area that has just been cleaned with a clean towel to preserve privacy. • If in a private room, keep the outside door closed, and if they are in a shared room, fully draw the curtain around the area before bathing.

Mobility and Support

CNAs and HHAs will encounter patients with a variety of mobility issues. Some will only need assistance for moving a long distance, and others may not be able to stand at all. There are several different devices and procedures that can aid a patient in moving or supporting themselves in their daily lives. The purpose of these devices and procedures is not only to move the patient but also to keep them as safe as possible. However, these devices and procedures are also meant to keep CNAs and HHAs safe from straining or injuring themselves when moving patients.

Here are a couple of things to practice when moving a patient:

- Lift with your legs, not your back.
- Request help whenever necessary.
- Clarify the procedure with the patient and explain how they may be able to help.
- Keep the patient close for good support and balance.
- Use a gait belt whenever it is necessary. (*See Lifts and Belts*)

Ambulation

Ambulation means being able to walk without caretaker assistance. Often, patients will require some assistance from a CNA or HHA to walk safely. For example, a patient who is weak on one side of their body will require support on that side. Other patients who can walk more independently may only require the CNA or HHA to walk behind them and be ready to assist if necessary. A CNA or HHA should act fast if a patient begins to fall and should guide the patient to fall backwards toward the CNA or HHA, as this will result in less injury and will help reduce the impact of the fall. The CNA or HHA should guide the patient toward a seat to allow them to rest before continuing to ambulate.

Patients may also use a variety of ambulatory devices to help them walk, and the device a patient uses depends on their unassisted walking ability. For example, a patient who doesn't need much help may use a cane, while a patient who requires a lot of assistance with walking may use a walker.

The table below includes several common ambulatory devices and a description of each:

Common Ambulatory Devices

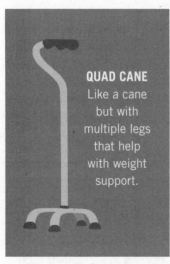

QUAD CANE
Like a cane but with multiple legs that help with weight support.

CANE
Helps with balance and weight support. Typically made from either wood or aluminum.

WALKER
A standard four-legged walker with a rubber tip at the end of each leg. Very stable and best suited for patients with slow-paced walking.

FRONT-WHEELED WALKER
Like a walker but with wheels on the two front legs. Useful for patients with a faster walking speed or those who can't lift a standard walker.

FOUR-WHEELED WALKER
Helps with balance but not with weight support. Best for patients who enjoy walking and can support their own body weight.

Lifts and Belts

In addition to assisting with walking, CNAs and HHAs also utilize different lifts and belts to help move a patient efficiently and safely from one point to another. This movement could involve helping a patient shift around in bed, assisting a patient to move up a flight of stairs, or any other mobility needs. There are a few common lifts and belts that all CNAs and HHAs should know how to safely operate.

Gait belt—This is a type of **transfer belt** that a patient wears to enable the CNA or HHA to help them ambulate or transfer from one position to another (sitting to standing, for example). The CNA or HHA secures the gait belt around the patient's waist over their clothes and grips the gait belt as the patient stands and walks. This belt gives the CNA or HHA something to hold on to that is not the patient's body or clothing, ensuring the patient's comfort and safety when ambulating or transferring.

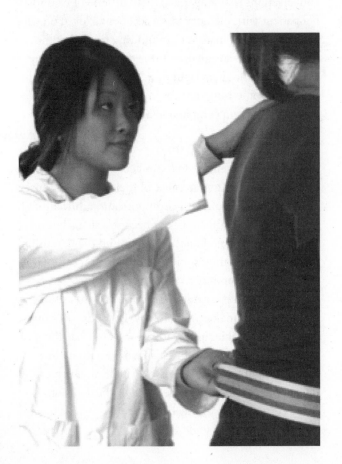

Chair lift—This lift is used to help a patient travel up or down a set of stairs. The patient should sit in the chair with both the armrests and footrests in the down position and buckle the safety belt provided. Most chair lifts have a simple one- or two-button 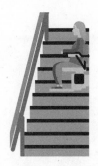 operation. Pressing and holding the button will move the chair lift up the stairs, and it will automatically stop at the top. Once safely at the top, the patient can be unbuckled from the safety belt and helped out of the chair. The patient and CNA or HHA should follow the same procedure to move down the stairs.

Hoyer lift—This lift is used to mechanically lift a patient in and out of a bed and could be used to place them into a wheelchair or bathtub. The CNA or HHA positions the patient's body in 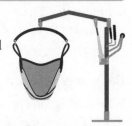 the sling and then uses the controls to lift and move the patient. Because of the difficulty and potential danger of using this device, only use the Hoyer lift when two staff members are available to assist. Also, use compassion with patients when using a Hoyer lift because they are at the mercy of the staff moving them and may become afraid or nervous about the process.

Medical trapeze bar—This bar hangs above the bed and is usually either connected to the head or foot of the bed or connected to the wall or ceiling. Patients use it for 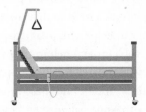 repositioning in bed and transferring in and out of bed. It is specifically useful for patients who are weak on one side of their body and can use their stronger side to leverage their body weight and help them move.

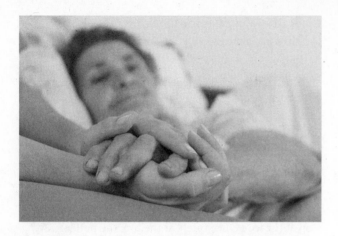

Caring for Patients with Memory Loss

There will be times that a CNA and HHA will need to care for a patient that has conditions that will impact their memory. These patients need to be treated with compassion and patience and should always be actively listened to.

Daily Interaction

When caring for a patient with memory loss, you should first **announce your entrance** to the patient's room and introduce yourself. Be friendly and speak as clearly as possible. Patients with memory loss are often easily startled and scared, and your announcements help them feel more prepared for your arrival. Always provide a patient with memory loss with simple and clear instructions. Keep instructions for the patient short and simple and be sure to include the patient's name. For example: "Mr. Smith, please place your cup on this table." Provide patients with only a **few decisions** at a time so that they are not overwhelmed and try to help them **problem solve** by understanding their problems and helping to overcome them. Sometimes, issues related to a lack of problem solving can result in frustrations, and these problems can easily be overcome with some patience and understanding.

Demeanor

When the patient speaks, it is important to be an **active listener**. Listening to the patient is vital because it helps them feel understood and enables the CNA or HHA to learn more about them. In every interaction, **remain calm and pleasant**. Since aides work so closely with patients, an aide's emotions can impact a patient's demeanor. Remaining composed while working, even when it can be frustrating or difficult, helps the patient feel respected and can greatly impact the quality of care provided. This positive **demeanor** can impact how patients feel about the quality of care and their willingness to accept assistance.

Acceptance

Patients with memory issues are often unaware of the time, year, or names of those around them, and they may even regress to a more childlike state. It is important to keep in mind that, even though they may seem childlike, they are adults who must be treated as such. It is cruel to try to get them to "act their age" or remember dates, names, and current events, and this type of treatment can cause frustration and anger. As a care provider, it is best to simply **accept their behaviors** and accommodate them as best you can without promoting additional or new behaviors. You can show your acceptance of the patient's behaviors by reframing conversations that may make them upset. For example, if a patient with memory loss asks about a loved on who has passed away, instead of reminding them that the family member has died, reframe the conversation by saying, "He's not here right now." By not reminding the patient of something that could cause them pain, you are showing them compassion and acceptance.

Distraction

Residents with memory loss can become paranoid and delusional, sometimes because of their declining senses and their frustration with communication difficulties. When a patient hallucinates or becomes suspicious of those around them, do not try to ground them, remind them that something is not real, or encourage the delusion by pretending to see the same thing. The best course of action is **casual distraction** towards a topic or activity that makes them happy. For some patients, talking about babies and children will improve their mood. You could also suggest a favorite activity like going outdoors or watching a favorite film. Distracting the patient can often pull them out of the delusion or redirect their energy away from their suspicions toward a more lighthearted topic.

MINI-QUIZ: ADLs

> **Directions:** Read each question below and choose the correct answer from the four choices provided. Only one choice is correct, so choose carefully.

1. A tool that hangs above the bed and is used by the patient to reposition themselves is called a

   A. Hoyer lift.

   B. trapeze bar.

   C. gait belt.

   D. transfer belt.

2. Which of the following helps promote resident dignity during personal hygiene?

   A. Provide denture adhesive.

   B. Complete care activities quickly so they are not late to breakfast.

   C. Select their clothes so they do not have to worry about them.

   D. Wake them up early so they are not rushed.

3. When using a Hoyer lift, you should always have

   A. one staff member with another on call.

   B. one staff member.

   C. two staff members.

   D. two staff members with another on call.

4. When a memory care resident is delusional, you should

   A. gently remind them of the correct day and time.

   B. provide them with items that help them reconnect with reality.

   C. join their delusion by pretending to see what they see.

   D. use casual distraction to change the subject.

5. Which of the following is NOT a basic ADL?

   A. Personal hygiene

   B. Ambulating

   C. Toileting

   D. Memory care.

6. An example of personal hygiene that falls outside of the CNA scope of practice is

   A. cutting nails.

   B. putting in dentures.

   C. shaving a beard.

   D. putting on glasses.

7. If you are completing a sponge bath in a double occupancy room, what should you do to preserve the dignity of the resident getting bathed?

   A. Cover them with a blanket as needed.

   B. Draw the curtain between the beds.

   C. Offer a bathrobe after you are finished.

   D. Shut the door to the entire room.

8. When walking a resident with a gait belt, where should you position yourself?

   A. In front of them in case they trip

   B. Behind them in case they fall

   C. Off to the side closest to the wall

   D. It does not matter.

9. Which of the following is an example of a physical comfort you can provide during bathing?

   A. Adjust the temperature of the water

   B. Use nice smelling candles

   C. Encourage conversation

   D. Allow time for the resident to soak and relax

10. Which of the following is NOT helpful when cleaning up after a toileting accident?

   A. Reminding the patient that they need to call you first next time

   B. Being discreet as you clean up so you do not draw attention to the accident

   C. Laying out clothing to help the resident change as needed

   D. Offering caring words of compassion as the resident may be upset

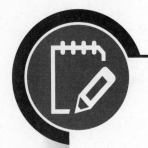

NOTES

ANSWER KEY AND EXPLANATIONS

1. B	3. C	5. D	7. B	9. A
2. A	4. D	6. A	8. B	10. A

1. **The correct answer is B.** A trapeze bar is a tool that hangs above the bed for the patient to reposition themselves. A Hoyer lift (choice A) is used to transfer an immobile patient. A gait belt and transfer belt (choices C and D) are used to help residents who cannot bear weight during transfers and ambulation.

2. **The correct answer is A.** Providing denture adhesive encourages the resident to wear their dentures, which promotes dignity. Completing care activities quickly (choice B) and selecting their clothes (choice C) benefits staff but can make the residents feel less dignified. Waking them up early (choice D) can be considered rude.

3. **The correct answer is C.** Two staff members are always required when using a Hoyer lift, as the patient is completely off the ground and could fall out. One staff member (choice A) and one staff member with another on call (choice B) are not safe options. Two staff members with another on call (choice D) may be necessary for some patients but is not required for all.

4. **The correct answer is D.** Casual distraction is a great tool when dealing with delusion among memory care patients. Reminding them of the day and time (choice A) and trying to help them reconnect with reality (choice B) can result in violent behaviors or added confusion. Joining their delusion (choice C) could increase the problem, not solve it.

5. **The correct answer is D.** Memory care is not a basic ADL, but there will be times that a memory care patient needs help with an ADL. Personal hygiene (choice A), ambulating (choice B), and toileting (choice C) are all basic ADLs.

6. **The correct answer is A.** Cutting toenails falls to a nurse or doctor as it can be done incorrectly and cause medical problems. In addition, some illnesses, such as diabetes, require specific foot care. Putting in dentures (choice B), shaving a beard (choice C), and putting on glasses (choice D) are all within the scope of practice for a CNA.

7. **The correct answer is B.** The curtain should be drawn between the beds so the other resident cannot see what you are doing. Covering them with a blanket (choice A) or shutting the door to the room itself (choice D) only allows some privacy, but there is still a roommate present. Offering a bathrobe (choice C) is nice, but the resident is still exposed during the bath.

8. **The correct answer is B.** When assisting someone with ambulation, you want to be behind them in case they trip or fall. You can guide them with the gait belt and allow your body to catch their fall if needed. You should never walk in front of them (choice A) or on the side by the wall (choice C) as these are unstable locations for the resident. It does matter where you position yourself (choice D).

9. **The correct answer is A.** Adjusting the temperature of the water is a physical comfort as it affects them physically. Encouraging conversation (choice C) and allowing time to soak and relax (choice D) are mental comforts. Candles are never allowed in a facility (choice B), and if they are used in a home, they provide mental comfort as well.

10. **The correct answer is A.** Immediately following a toileting accident is NOT the time to remind the resident to ask for help as this is very demeaning and does not promote dignity. Choices B, C, and D all focus on patient dignity first to care for the whole person and not just the toileting mess.

NUTRITION

Nutrition involves how we obtain nutrients that we need for health, usually through consuming food or liquids. As a CNA or HHA, it is important to understand the importance of nutrition in patient health and wellbeing. Patients under the care of medical professionals often require specific amounts of vitamins and nutrients to keep their bodies as healthy as possible, and others require meals prepared in a specific way that will enable them to consume their meals.

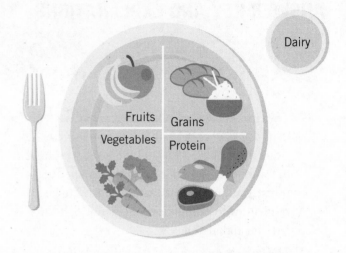

To ensure that a patient receives proper nutrition, it is important to understand the five main food groups and how they contribute to overall health. Balancing these food groups ensures that patients receive the right number of vitamins and nutrients to keep their bodies and minds healthy. Because patients have varying needs concerning nutrition, it is also important for a CNA and HHA to understand the different types of diets and the different eating complications they may encounter. Some patients may need their food cut, blended, or chopped in a particular way to make it safe to eat, and some patients may have trouble swallowing, chewing, or feeding themselves. The CNA or HHA should be aware of these issues related to patient nutrition in order to provide care that will keep the patient safe and healthy.

Five Main Food Groups

Portioning the five main food groups is an important part of preparing any meal. All meals should be portioned so that fruits and vegetables, grains, protein, and dairy make it onto the plate. This allows for the necessary vitamins, minerals, and other nutrients to make it into the digestive system to promote a healthy body. But we need a greater amount of food from some food groups over others, so portions on a plate from each food group will not be equal in size. For instance, because our bodies require more nutrients found in fruits and vegetables, the food portions on a prepared plate should contain more fruits and vegetables than the other food subgroups.

Exceptions to this portioning are made if an individual has an allergy of some kind or cannot chew or digest a certain type of food. Adjustments can be made for these exceptions, but it is important that the substitutions hold similar nutrients, or the individual takes supplements that will give them the missing nutrients.

Types of Diets

Medical diet types have been developed to accommodate patients that are unable to eat certain foods due to allergies or physical inability. There are many different types of reasons that a patient needs to be on a specific diet type, but the diet types we will discuss will be based on physical needs. Some patients might lack the physical ability to chew, swallow, or digest certain foods; thus, they require a special type of diet.

On the following page is a table indicating the most common diet types in healthcare, what patient conditions they are used for, the texture of the diet type, and what they typically consist of.

Diabetic Diets

Diabetic patients need to carefully watch their diets to make sure they are receiving enough nutrients while limiting glucose that their body cannot process effectively. With this type of diet, patients need to avoid sugar and processed sweets. A patient's meal schedule determines the amount of insulin they receive each day. Foods that are within those meals should be as healthy as possible, and diabetic patients should try to avoid having too much saturated or trans fats, sodium, and cholesterol. It is important to guide patients towards sugar-free options whenever possible.

Simple carbohydrates like white bread, potatoes, candy, and cookies are quick energy sources that bodies break down quickly. They can cause blood sugar to spike. But complex carbohydrates, like whole grain breads, pastas, sweet potatoes and beans take longer to break down and have less of an effect on your blood sugar levels than simple carbohydrates.

Caring for Patients with Nutrition Complications

There are many factors that can cause an individual to refuse or be unable to eat a nutritional diet. A few of these factors have already been mentioned in this chapter, including a patient's inability to consume food, having food allergies, or needing a special diet for physical reasons. Any factors that cause a patient not to receive essential food or nutrients should be addressed so that they are able to do so. Patients who require nutritional and feeding assistance should always be treated with compassion and patience. It is important to try to preserve their dignity when assisting them; for some, it is their first time needing assistance with a task like eating a meal.

MOST COMMON MEDICAL DIET TYPES			
DIET TYPE	USED FOR	FOOD TEXTURE	CONSISTS OF
Regular diet	Fully capable patients who have no problems chewing, swallowing, or digesting.	Varying textures of foods from all five food groups.	Anything that the patient is not allergic to; no modifications are made.
Soft diet	Transitional diet between a liquid diet and a regular diet. Common after surgery or injury.	Softer foods that can still be chewed.	Fish, lean meats, liquids, potatoes, and soft breads.
Mechanical soft diet	Patients who have trouble chewing. Common diet for a patient who has had a stroke or dental issues like missing teeth; this type of diet is one step away from a liquid diet and toward a regular diet.	Chopped, ground, or puréed.	Any kind of food that has been mechanically processed to drastically reduce the chewing needed.
Puréed diet	Patients who have physical difficulty chewing or have lost the cognitive ability to understand that chewing is necessary (such as with Alzheimer's disease).	Strictly puréed.	Puréed foods that do not require chewing. Examples are mashed potatoes or a smoothie. Every food, including meats, vegetables, fruits, and grains, can and should be offered in this form if the patient enjoys it.
Liquid diet	Patients who have trouble chewing or need to reduce residue in the GI tract.	High liquid content or, at times, strictly liquid.	Includes soups, juice, creamed cereals, and even eggs if the patient can swallow and/or tolerate them.

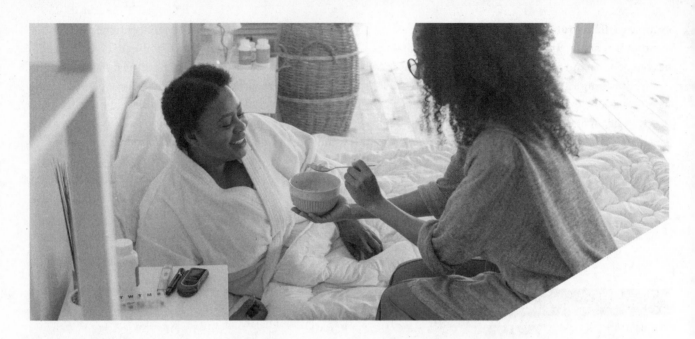

Inability to Chew, Swallow, or Digest

If a patient has trouble consuming food, they can become discouraged. Some may even avoid asking for help as it may make them feel inferior. The best way to empower them is to give them a diet that is easier to consume. In addition, staff observance or physical assistance may be needed, but this assistance should be offered in the most gentle and positive manner possible to preserve the dignity of the patient.

Physical Inability to Feed

Similar to patients who have trouble consuming food, patients who have difficulty feeding themselves can become discouraged. If you observe this, you may recommend a patient for occupational therapy, which can help them to use assistive tools such as modified spoons and cups to maximize their independence. If all else fails, a patient may require your physical assistance to help them consume their food, but this should be used as a last resort after all modifications have been attempted. A resident may not be able to feed themselves quickly, but that does not mean they should be stripped of their independence. Make sure they are provided with any necessary modified tools (spoons, forks, cups etc.) as specified in their care plan.

Memory or Cognitive Impairment

Patients with memory loss will sometimes forget to eat. Sticking to a meal schedule where a healthcare professional can observe them eating is a good way to address this. In addition, some memory-impaired patients may forget the food consumption process and will benefit from cues during each meal. On top of that, some foods can induce memory loss in a patient, and they should be placed on a diet limiting those foods. For example, processed cheeses and meats have been known to negatively affect patients who have Alzheimer's disease.

Cultural Restrictions

There are many cultures in the world that place restrictions on the consumption of certain types of food. To help patients adhere to these restrictions, they should be put on a diet that does not contain any of these foods and offers nutrient-dense substitutions in their place.

Observe Nonverbal Patients

Nonverbal patients express their needs without using words. Headshaking, tightening facial muscles, flailing hands, and head-turning are all nonverbal cues that the patient does not like what is being offered or the way it is being offered. If you observe any of these behaviors, ask yes/no clarifying questions to get to the root of their frustration.

MINI-QUIZ: NUTRITION

Directions: Read each question below and choose the correct answer from the four choices provided. Only one choice is correct, so choose carefully.

1. Which of the following food groups should be the most represented on a regular diet patient's plate?

   A. Dairy

   B. Protein

   C. Fruits and vegetables

   D. Grains

2. Which type of diet is recommended for someone with dental pain?

   A. Soft

   B. Mechanical soft

   C. Puréed

   D. Liquid

3. Which of the following foods cannot be included in a puréed diet?

   A. Meat

   B. Coconut

   C. Broccoli

   D. Pasta

4. Which of the following is unsafe in a liquid diet?

   A. Cookie milkshake

   B. Carbonated soda

   C. Honey

   D. Butter

5. Which type of therapist can assist in helping a resident with feeding tools?

   A. Physical

   B. Occupational

   C. Respiratory

   D. Speech

6. Patients on which type of diet can consume hard cheeses without modification?

   A. Soft

   B. Mechanical soft

   C. Puréed

   D. Regular

7. When a nonverbal resident turns their head away when a particular food is presented, they might

   A. dislike the food.

   B. feel excited.

   C. feel fatigued.

   D. be attempting to turn toward the food.

8. Is butter allowed in a liquid diet?

   A. No, it is forbidden.

   B. Yes, but only if it's melted.

   C. Yes, but only in moderation.

   D. Yes, it does not require any modifications.

9. Which of the following is the most restrictive type of staff-related assistance?

   A. Setting up the meal tray and utensils

   B. Providing verbal cues to keep eating

   C. Providing physical touch cues to bring the fork to the mouth

   D. Assisting by lifting a cup up to the mouth

10. Which of the following is not permitted for those on a modified diet?

    A. Peanut butter

    B. Lettuce

    C. Rice

    D. Honey

ANSWER KEY AND EXPLANATIONS

1. C	3. B	5. B	7. A	9. D
2. B	4. A	6. D	8. B	10. B

1. **The correct answer is C.** Fruits and vegetables (with an emphasis on vegetables) should make up roughly 50% of the plate. The other 50% should be a combination of protein (choice B) and grains (choice D). Dairy (choice A) can be added but should be limited in comparison.

2. **The correct answer is B.** A mechanical soft diet is the best type of diet for dental pain. A soft diet (choice A) may require too much chewing. Puréed (choice C) and liquid (choice D) diets may work, but they are extreme choices that should be prescribed by a dentist if needed.

3. **The correct answer is B.** Coconut cannot be properly puréed, thus making it impossible for inclusion within this diet. Meat (choice A), broccoli (choice B), and pasta (choice D) can all be puréed to a safe consistency and SHOULD be included in this type of diet.

4. **The correct answer is A.** The cookie component of the milkshake is not safe on a liquid diet. However, soda (choice B), honey (choice C) and even butter (choice D) are all permitted.

5. **The correct answer is B.** Occupational therapists work with patients to analyze their physical needs during feeding. Assistive devices such as modified spoons and cups can help the patient retain their independence. The other therapists (choices A, C, and D) do not work in this arena.

6. **The correct answer is D.** Hard cheeses, such as parmesan, can only be consumed without modification on a regular diet. All other diets (choices A, B, and C) require modifications or have hard cheese restrictions.

7. **The correct answer is A.** Turning their head away from a particular food is often a clear indication that a nonverbal resident does not like it. Excitement (choice B) and fatigue (choice C) are often accompanied by other sounds and movements. Trying to turn toward the food (choice D) could be possible, but it would not be limited to only one type of food.

8. **The correct answer is B.** Butter is a vital fat that can fortify a liquid diet, but it needs to be melted. It is not forbidden (choice A). It does not need to be restricted unless a patient has other health issues like heart disease (choice C), but it does require modification (choice D).

9. **The correct answer is D.** Any type of full-on physical assistance is the most restrictive type of assistance as it takes away the patient's right to independence. Setting up the meal tray and utensils (choice A) is done for all patients. Providing verbal cues (choice B) and physical touch cues (choice C) allow for more independence than physically lifting the cup to their mouth.

10. **The correct answer is B.** Lettuce cannot be mechanically modified or puréed and does not come in a liquid form; thus, it is only safe within a regular diet. Peanut butter (choice A) is only restricted on a liquid diet. Rice (choice C) and honey (choice D) are both able to be modified for all diet types.

BODY MECHANICS AND RANGE OF MOTION

Body mechanics are the ways an individual carries or holds themselves, and **range of motion** is the movement capability of a body's specific joint. There are many factors to consider when caring for patients, but some of the most fundamental ways CNAs and HHAs interact with a patient happens in ADLs involving the mechanics and range of the human body.

A human body's mechanics and range of motion dictate that body's abilities, and each body's mechanics and range are unique in their own ways. Each joint in the human body has a different range of motion, and everyone has their own level of ability to bend each joint. Therefore, during physical therapy or similar exercises, it is important to know the physical ability of a patient's body when performing actions like moving a limb away from the body, called **abducting**, or moving a limb toward the body, called **adducting**.

Using proper body mechanics helps to protect the patient and the staff from injury and should be practiced by everyone, including the patient's family. A CNA or HHA should know their own body's limits when assisting a patient with getting out of bed, walking, and standing. Knowing your body's limits, taking proper precautions, and properly using the tools available to promote safe movement can help a CNA, HHA, or family member move a patient without injury.

Any range of motion exercises prescribed by a doctor or therapist will be shown to you specifically and will also come with a handout to help ensure that you complete the activities correctly to avoid injury to the patient.

Comfort and Safety

The comfort of a patient is dependent on body mechanics and range of motion when relative to the patient's posture, position, limitations, or unique conditions. For example, a bed-bound patient should be repositioned every two hours to maximize comfort and minimize the chance of bed sores forming. Another good example of positioning a patient for comfort is if a patient experiences pain in one shoulder, then they should rest on their back or other shoulder to try and reduce the pain. Practicing proper use of body mechanics and range of motion exercises will keep patients, family, and staff safe during the various tasks performed in healthcare facilities. Negligence to do so can result in both minor and major injuries to the musculoskeletal system, with many requiring lengthy recoveries.

Here are a few examples of potential injuries:

Potential Injuries

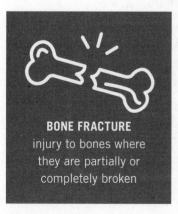

BONE FRACTURE
injury to bones where they are partially or completely broken

SPRAIN
stress to the joint that can overstretch or tear the ligaments

STRAIN
tearing of muscle fibers, commonly caused by over-stretching

RUPTURE
partial or complete tear in a tendon

TISSUE DAMAGE
damage to ligaments, tendons, and muscles throughout the body

Bed Sores

Bed sores are a common injury caused not by movement but by lack of movement. They appear from laying or sitting in one place for a long period of time. The patient's body position when lying or sitting can impact how the sore develops.

Here are the four stages of bed sores:

STAGE 1

Warm to the touch with some redness

STAGE 2

An open sore, blister, or scrape with a discolored area

STAGE 3

Crater-like appearance due to damage below the skin's surface

STAGE 4

Serious damage with a large wound resulting in skin and tissue loss (These have the highest chance of becoming infected.)

Positions and Postures

Body mechanics includes the way someone carries or holds their body, and a patient's **position** and **posture** dictate how their body is oriented when supporting or moving themselves. There are multiple positions and postures that the human body can maintain.

Here are the three main positions used in healthcare:

- **Supine**—patient lying on their back.
- **Prone**—patient lying on their stomach.
- **Lateral**—patient lying on their side.

Posture involves how someone supports their body while sitting or standing. A patient's posture can impact their ability to move in different ways. If a patient's posture is not correct, then issues and injuries can result. Factors like the shape of a patient's spine and their muscle strength can impact posture.

Here are some postures that are commonly referenced in healthcare:

- **Static posture**—standing, sitting, or lying down; called *static* because this posture involves support, not movement.
- **Dynamic posture**—moving; how a patient supports their body while in motion.
- **Kyphosis posture**—curved shoulders; creates excessive curving of the back.
- **Lordosis posture**—excessive curvature of the lower part of the spine; can tilt the pelvis past a normal point.

Ambulation and Movement

Dynamic posture, the posture of movement, has a large effect on how well a patient moves, including their ability to walk. Oftentimes, you may encounter patients with limps, spinal problems, or other conditions impacting posture. This can directly affect the ability to ambulate. **Ambulation** is the ability to walk with or without an aid. Devices such as gait belts and walkers are common tools used to help a patient walk to a destination.

When helping a patient walk or move, an aide should

always consider their body mechanics and range of motion. If an aide bends, pulls, or pushes a patient into a position that their body cannot handle, injuries can occur. These injuries could be temporary, or they could negatively affect a current condition. Aides can help prevent injuries by utilizing correct body mechanics and range of motion guidelines and correct lifting/moving techniques and equipment. Using correct procedures and tools also protects staff from injuries related to ambulation tasks.

Range of Motion

Patients perform **range of motion (ROM)** exercises for recovery after an injury or surgery and to maintain the maximum range of usage for muscles and joints, even as a person ages.

- **Active ROM**—completed by the patient without any assistance from the CNA.
- **Active Assisted ROM**—completed by the patient with limited assistance from the CNA.
- **Passive ROM**—completed by the CNA with little to no assistance from the patient. This is often for patients who cannot physically or cognitively participate.

The following images show examples of some common ROM exercises:

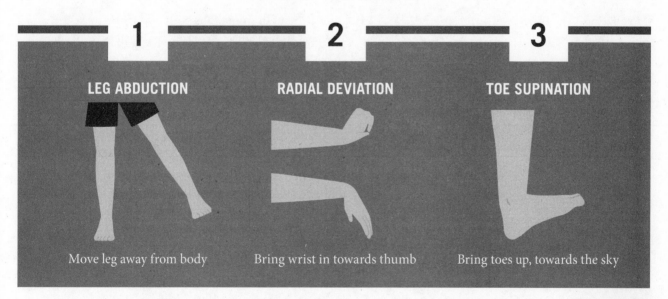

ROM Exercises

1	2	3
LEG ABDUCTION	**RADIAL DEVIATION**	**TOE SUPINATION**
Move leg away from body	Bring wrist in towards thumb	Bring toes up, towards the sky

Always tell the resident to report any pain or discomfort IMMEDIATELY and stop if they report either of these. In addition, any concerns during ROM exercises should be both documented and reported to the nurse.

Range of Motion Vocabulary

Depending on a patient's needs, the requested ROM activities will vary. There are eight main types of ROM exercises that are important to know. Those exercises are listed below with some common exercise examples:

COMMON EXERCISE EXAMPLES		
TERM	**DEFINITION**	**EXAMPLE**
Adduction	bring together	Fingers of the hand spread wide apart, bringing them together at the center of the hand
Abduction	spread apart	Standing straight with hands at sides of the body, swinging hands from sides of the body up toward shoulders
Flexion	bend	Holding arm straight out from the body with palm toward ceiling, bending at elbow joint until hand is near ear
Extension	extend	Sitting in a chair with feet flat on the floor, straightening knee joint until in a standing position
Pronation	turn down to the ground	Holding arm out in front of the body with palm toward the ceiling, rotating at the wrist until palm faces the floor
Supination	turn up to the sky	Sitting with foot flat on the floor, keeping the heel of the foot on the ground and lifting the toes toward the ceiling
Internal/ external rotation	twist, turn, or rotate. (*Internal* means "towards the body"; *external* means "away from the body")	Internal rotation: While standing, twist hip joint inward until thigh and toes point toward center of body. External rotation: While standing with toes and thigh pointing toward center of body, twist outward at hip joint until thigh and toes point away from body
Deviation	the same as flexion or adduction, but focuses on the radial bones and joints	With hand extended in front of the body, bend at wrist joint toward the ceiling and then toward the floor
Opposition	bring the tip of the thumb to the pads of the other fingers	With palm facing the ceiling, touch the thumb to the index finger and then back to the neutral position, repeat with all fingers

MINI-QUIZ: BODY MECHANICS AND RANGE OF MOTION

Directions: Read each question below and choose the correct answer from the four choices provided. Only one choice is correct, so choose carefully.

1. Which of the following injuries is commonly caused by overstretching?

   A. Sprain

   B. Fracture

   C. Strain

   D. Rupture

2. If a resident is assigned a finger adduction exercise, they are being asked to

   A. spread their fingers apart.

   B. bring their fingers together.

   C. tap each finger with their thumb.

   D. rotate their wrist.

3. If a resident is ordered to lay prone, what position are they in?

   A. On their stomach facing down

   B. On their back facing up

   C. On their side with legs bent

   D. On their side with legs straight

4. The technical term for normal posture while moving is_____ posture.

   A. static

   B. kyphosis

   C. lordosis

   D. dynamic

5. Which of the following stages of bedsores results in serious tissue damage?

   A. Stage 3

   B. Stage 2

   C. Stage 4

   D. Stage 1

6. If a ROM exercise is completely done by the patient, it is called a(n) _____ ROM.

   A. active

   B. active assisted

   C. passive

   D. independent

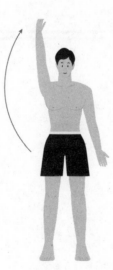

7. Based on this image, what is this ROM called?

   A. Pronation of the arm

   B. Supination of the arm

   C. Flexion of the arm

   D. Extension of the arm

8. If a patient reports discomfort during ROM exercises, it is the responsibility of the CNA to

   A. speak words of encouragement.

   B. skip over that ROM.

   C. have them try it again slowly.

   D. stop the ROM and report it to the nurse.

9. A CNA is directed to provide passive range of motion for a resident that recently had a hip replacement. Which of the following is the best example of this task?

   A. The CNA has the patient rotate their hip as they count their reps.

   B. The CNA shows the patient how to rotate their hip and then allows them to do it themselves.

   C. The CNA manually rotates the hip for 10 reps.

   D. The CNA asks the patient to extend and flex their toes.

10. Which of the following is NOT an example of an assistive device?

    A. Wheelchair seat belt

    B. Cane

    C. Braces

    D. Splints

NOTES

ANSWER KEY AND EXPLANATIONS

1. C	3. A	5. C	7. B	9. C
2. B	4. D	6. A	8. D	10. A

1. **The correct answer is C.** A strain is a tear that is often caused by overstretching something, either voluntarily or by accident. Sprains (choice A), fractures (choice B), and ruptures (choice D) are not common injuries related to overstretching.

2. **The correct answer is B.** Adduction is the act of coming together. Spreading their fingers apart (choice A) would be called abduction. Tapping each finger with their thumb (choice C) is called opposition. Rotating their wrist (choice D) is called radial deviation.

3. **The correct answer is A.** A prone position is lying flat on your stomach facing down. When you are on your back facing up (choice B), you are supine. When you are on your side, (choices C and D) you are lateral.

4. **The correct answer is D.** Dynamic posture is the term for normal posture while moving. Static posture (choice A) is when you are remaining still. Kyphosis posture (choice B) is when the shoulders are curved, and lordosis posture (choice C) is when the bottom of the spine is curved.

5. **The correct answer is C.** Stage 4 bedsores (choice C) result in skin damage and tissue damage below the skin; there is usually extensive damage with a large wound and tissue loss in addition to the skin. Stage 1 bedsores (choice D) are warm to the touch and have redness. Stage 2 bedsores (choice B) do have an open sore, blister, or scrape and the area may be discolored, but underlying tissue is not damaged. Stage 3 bedsores (choice A) result in a crater-like appearance due to damage below the skin's surface.

6. **The correct answer is A.** Active ROM means the exercise is done entirely by the patient. Active assisted ROM (choice B) requires minimal assistance from staff. Passive ROM (choice C) requires full assistance from staff. Independent ROM (choice D) is not a medical term and is not used.

7. **The correct term is B.** The arm is moving up towards the sky, which is called supination. Pronation of the arm (choice A) would be moving towards the floor. Flexion of the arm (choice C) would be bending at the elbow or bringing it in close to the midline. Extension of the arm (choice D) would be extending it away from the body.

8. **The correct answer is D.** Any report of discomfort by the resident during ROM exercises should result in stopping the activity and reporting it to the nurse. You will get guidance from there. It is outside of the CNA's scope of practice to speak words of encouragement (choice A), skip over a ROM (choice B), or have the patient try it again slowly (choice C) without direct guidance from the nurse or physical therapist.

9. **The correct answer is C.** Passive range of motion requires the CNA to do the work and not the patient. Choices A and D are examples of active range of motion. Choice B is an example of assisted active range of motion.

10. **The correct answer is A.** An assistive device helps to make a task easier to perform. A wheelchair seat belt increases safety but is a form of restraint. A cane (choice B), braces (choice C), and splints (choice D) are all examples of assistive devices as they increase the ease of walking.

THE AGING PROCESS

During **the aging process**, body systems go through changes, and older people tend to lose some of the body functions once provided through the five senses. As a CNA or HHA, it is important to understand the aging process so your expectations when helping elders match their unique aging processes. Being aware of the changes people generally go through as they age can help CNAs and HHAs avoid potential harm like infections or falls and support patients through proper transfer procedures and use of assistive devices. Aides should also be aware that, as elders lose some skills, their bodies naturally make up for them with other senses. Being aware of the complexity of the aging process and how it uniquely affects each individual can help a CNA or HHA care for their elderly patients with compassion and skill.

Body Systems

The aging process happens slowly and gradually over time, affecting multiple systems in a myriad of ways. It is helpful to think of aging as a marathon. The human body did not develop quickly; thus, the aging of the human body also occurs over time. Even so, there are some common processes that happen as the body ages.

As someone goes through the aging process, their maximum organ functions decrease as cells divide slower and waste builds up. In the heart, walls become thicker, and aorta lose flexibility, making the heart less efficient with pumping blood. Heart rate is slower to return to normal after exertion. The number of neurons and connections between them in the brain and nervous system decrease.

Digestion takes longer as the production of digestive juices decreases. Body temperature becomes more difficult to regulate. Bones become weaker and can break more easily while joints stiffen, and muscle tissue loses strength. In the eyes, lenses can become cloudy with thicker irises and thinner retinas. Skin begins to lose elasticity, and eardrums become thicker. Hair becomes gray or white and slows in growth while nails become thinner and tend to break more easily.

Higher Risks

All areas of decline can cause a variety of issues. As a CNA or HHA, there are two main risks that could affect a person as they age that are important to understand: infections and falls. Your role as a CNA and HHA can help to decrease the likelihood of these related problems by helping the patient work through them should they arise.

Older patients are at a higher risk for **infections**. The slowdown in both cell production and organ function (as well as other losses) leads to a weakened immune system. To help older patients avoid infection, wash your hands before and after all care and keep their area and objects around them clean. Lots of germs exist in exceptionally high touch areas like their glasses, remote, and telephone, so make sure to thoroughly clean those areas to avoid spreading infection.

Due to a combination of decreased vision, stiff joints, weak muscles, and poor bone density, older patients are also at a higher risk for **falls**. Not only are they at higher risk for falls, but the likelihood that the fall will cause damage, such as a broken bone, is much higher. Be aware of fall risks in their area, and always practice safe transfer procedures to reduce the risk of falls. Fall risks may include uneven surfaces, clutter, or spills. The CNA or HHA should make sure that the area around a patient's bed and any area where they may be moving around is free of these hazards. Also ensure that the patient has any assistive devices that they may need, such as canes, walkers, or wheelchairs, and take all safety precautions when transferring them from one area to another, as discussed in the *Mobility and Support* section.

The Five Senses

The most evident and noticeable changes for the aging person occur across **the five senses**: sight, hearing, taste, smell, and touch. It is important for a CNA or HHA to know how aging affects each of the five senses so they can provide care and comfort. Remember that each patient is different, and the way their senses are affected will vary.

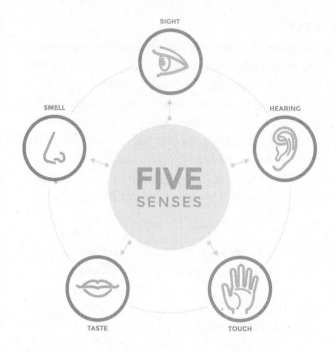

FIVE SENSES

SIGHT

SMELL

HEARING

TASTE

TOUCH

Sight

Losing quality in **eyesight** is one of the earliest changes related to aging and occurs in the mid-40s to early 50s. Some people notice changes earlier, while others do not experience vision changes until well into their 50s

or 60s. There are several common eye afflictions that an aide may encounter when working with an elderly patient. Any sudden change in eyesight requires medical attention, so note this in your documentation if a patient reports it.

The chart below presents several common sight-related terms and their effects.

Hearing

As the eardrum thickens and the ear canal thins, hearing decreases with age and is a common age-related decline. Most people experience at least a minor decrease in hearing as they age. Many older adults will require hearing aids at some point, and you, as their care provider, must ensure patients use their hearing aids.

For many elder patients, their first hearing issue involves **speech**. High-frequency words become difficult to hear, and a person may miss small sections of the conversation or require clarification on words that sound the same. Next, **background noise** can become an issue when its presence gets harder to filter. People with hearing loss do better with minimal background

COMMON SIGHT-RELATED TERMS	
TERM	**DEFINITION**
Presbyopia	decrease in the ability to see up close; results in the need for reading glasses.
Floaters	spots in vision; increase with age regardless of lighting.
Dry Eyes	when eye ducts produce too little or poor-quality tears. Replacement artificial tears can be helpful. Some medications and diseases may aggravate dry eyes.
Glaucoma	related to pressure behind the eye, leading to blindness if not treated in time; often onset in old age.
Age-related Macular Degeneration	deterioration of the macular (part of the retina); slowly cuts off vision, sometimes starting in the middle, leaving blind spots that increase over time.
Cataracts	cloudy spots on the lens of the eye; do not cause any pain or redness but affect vision because of lens fogginess.
Diabetic Retinopathy	can cause blindness; retinal damage when blood vessels are inefficient in delivering blood and nutrients. Symptoms can occur suddenly and include floaters and cloudiness. Annual eye exams with dilation are critical to catching this early.

noise, so turning off the T.V. or radio when giving instructions during care can help dramatically.

Eventually, some patients are only able to hear with assistance. This level of hearing loss requires that the person uses **hearing aids**, or those communicating with them must raise their voices to communicate, which is not respectful. If you work with a resident who has this level of hearing loss, have them assist you with putting in their hearing aids; this activity allows them to actively participate in conversation and respond to your instructions and questions. Do not wait until you have already dressed, transferred, and toileted them, as this has left them in silence through most of their cares.

Taste

The number of taste buds decreases with age, causing food preferences to shift and an increase in the use of seasoning to offset dull tastes. If a complete loss of taste occurs, chewing or swallowing can become compromised. A dramatic increase in the use of seasoning (such as salt) can also cause other health problems. Offer patients added seasonings that do not negatively affect the body, such as oregano, garlic, and onion powder.

Smell

Along with a decrease in taste, people who are aging also experience a decrease in their sense of smell as the two senses work together. More than half of all older adults report either a reduction in the ability to smell or, more commonly, a decrease in the ability to discriminate between smells. One way to assist residents is to announce the smells as you are heading to the cafeteria. This allows them time to take in the smell without being corrected for incorrectly identifying it.

Touch

Sensitivity to touch decreases with age due to poorer circulation and the inability to regulate body temperature. Hot and cold sensations decrease, and many people report being colder as they age, regardless of the outside temperature. To accommodate this, it is important to assist the resident in selecting clothing that allows for easy adjustment based on temperature, such as dressing in layers that can be removed or keeping a sweater nearby if they get cold. In addition, ensure that residents can wear non-slip socks or shoes to help keep heat in and cold out. When caring for a patient, make sure to be firm yet gentle in your touch to accommodate an older person's less sensitive touch receptors.

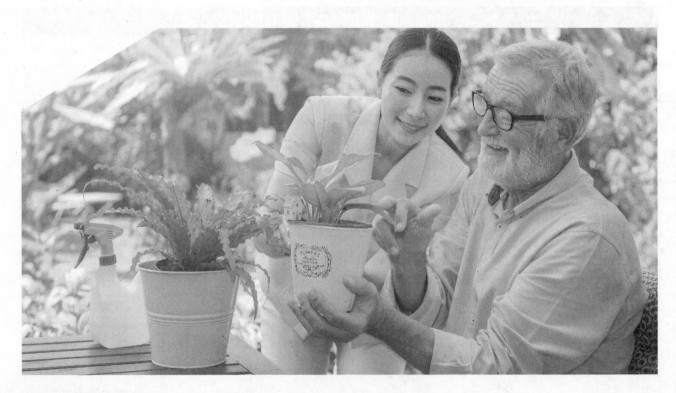

5

MINI-QUIZ: AGING PROCESS

Directions: Read each question below and choose the correct answer from the four choices provided. Only one choice is correct, so choose carefully.

1. A natural age-related vision problem is
   A. glaucoma.
   B. cataracts.
   C. age-related macular degeneration.
   D. presbyopia.

2. The process of slowly losing vision from the center of the pupil outward is called
   A. glaucoma.
   B. age-related macular degeneration.
   C. cataracts.
   D. diabetic retinopathy.

3. Age-related hearing loss is caused in part by
   A. the thickening of the eardrum.
   B. exposure to loud machinery during their working years.
   C. the thickening of the ear canal.
   D. a buildup of earwax.

4. One way to assist a resident who complains of a loss of taste is to
   A. adjust their menu to include spicier foods.
   B. encourage the use of salt.
   C. offer seasonings such as garlic and onion powder.
   D. pair up stronger flavors so the taste is more noticeable.

5. Age-related decline in touch includes
   A. heightened sensitivity.
   B. rough skin.
   C. dry skin.
   D. decreased sensitivity.

6. Which sense is directly connected with smell?
   A. Taste
   B. Vision
   C. Hearing
   D. Touch

7. Which of the following is NOT related to the aging process?
   A. Decrease in skin elasticity
   B. Increase in agitation
   C. Increase in waste buildup
   D. Decrease in cell growth

8. Which of the following is an age-related decline specific to your organs?
   A. Cells divide slower
   B. Joints stiffen
   C. Easy breakage
   D. Circulation slows down

9. Which of the following is a common digestion-related change as you age?
   A. Overproduction of digestive juices
   B. Inability to absorb nutrients
   C. Decrease in esophageal efficiency
   D. Underproduction of digestive juices

10. One way to help a resident with mild to moderate hearing loss is to
    A. speak loudly so they can hear you.
    B. recommend they use hearing aids.
    C. turn down the T.V. during cares.
    D. turn off the T.V. during cares.

ANSWER KEY AND EXPLANATIONS

1. D	**3.** A	**5.** D	**7.** B	**9.** D
2. B	**4.** C	**6.** A	**8.** A	**10.** D

1. **The correct answer is D.** Presbyopia is the difficulty to see up close, such as with reading. Glaucoma (Choice A), cataracts (choice B), and age-related macular degeneration (choice C) are all vision problems that are not naturally occurring in everyone as they age.

2. **The correct answer is B.** Age-related macular degeneration starts with blind spots in the center of your vision and works outward. Glaucoma (choice A) starts with peripheral vision loss. Cataracts (choice C) and diabetic retinopathy (choice D) start with cloudy vision.

3. **The correct answer is A.** With age, the eardrum thickens, which attributes to a natural decline in hearing. Loud machinery (choice B) can cause hearing loss, but it is not related to age. The ear canal thins, not thickens, with age (choice C), and a buildup of earwax (choice D) can cause hearing loss at any age.

4. **The correct answer is C.** Offering seasonings such as garlic and onion powder allows the resident to increase the flavor without health repercussions. The use of added salt (choice B) can negatively affect their health. Adding spicier foods (choice A) or more pungent food pairings (choice D) may not help the resident and may cause stomach upset.

5. **The correct answer is D.** Decreased sensitivity occurs due to a decrease in circulation and the ability to regulate body temperature. Heightened sensitivity (choice A) is not related to age. Rough skin (choice B) and dry skin (choice C) are not related to age and can occur at any age.

6. **The correct answer is A.** Taste and smell are directly connected. Your sense of smell transmits signals to your mouth, thus preparing you for the taste of an expected food. Vision (choice B), hearing (choice C), and touch (choice D) are not directly connected with smell.

7. **The correct answer is B.** Increase in agitation is not related to the aging process, although some people report this. A decrease in skin elasticity (choice A), cell growth (choice D), and an increase in waste buildup (choice C) are all related to the aging process.

8. **The correct answer is A.** Cells divide slower within organs due to age. Joints do stiffen (choice B), bones break easier (choice C), and circulation slows down (choice D), but these are not organ related.

9. **The correct answer is D.** With age comes an underproduction of digestive juices from the respective organs, which leads to a slower overall digestion. The body is still able to absorb nutrients (choice B) and the esophagus does not automatically decrease in efficiency (choice C). Overproduction of digestive juices (choice A) is not related specifically to age.

10. **The correct answer is D.** Turning off the T.V. during cares eliminates additional background noise that can make hearing difficult for those with mild to moderate hearing loss. Speaking loudly (choice A) and recommending hearing aids (choice B) are both disrespectful to the resident. Turning down the T.V. can make it even harder to hear, as the background noise is not eliminated but is too low to distinguish clearly.

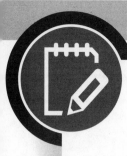

NOTES

SUMMING IT UP

- Activities of Daily Living (ADLs) are the daily physical needs that people have that are necessary for a healthy state of living and include tasks like ambulating, dressing, personal hygiene, feeding, continence, toileting, and bathing.

- The Katz Index is a questionnaire checklist used to determine if a patient can or cannot independently perform basic ADLs.

- When making decisions with and for the patient about care, a CNA or HHA should always keep safety and dignity at the forefront of ADL plans and procedures.

  o To preserve patient safety, a CNA or HHA should avoid accidents, follow proper body movements, take precautions with food and liquids, clean the patient's body in a safe order, and avoid cutting toenails.

  o A CNA or HHA can preserve patient dignity through communication, honoring patient preferences, listening to family input, following the patient's care plan, and using discretion.

- CNAs and HHAs will encounter patients with a variety of mobility issues.

  o Ambulation means being able to walk without caretaker assistance. Often, patients will require some assistance from a CNA or HHA to walk safely.

  o Patients may also use a variety of ambulatory devices to help them walk like canes or walkers.

  o Lifts and belts help move patients from one point to another, such as a Hoyer lift, chair lift, trapeze bar, or gait belt.

- When caring for a patient with memory loss, a CNA or HHA should announce their entrance, give simple and clear instructions, allow the patient to make a few decisions, help the patient to problem solve, be an active listener, remain calm and pleasant with a positive demeanor, accept their patient's behaviors, and casually distract the patient when necessary.

- Nutrition involves how we obtain nutrients that we need for health, usually through consuming food or liquids.

- The five food groups are fruits, vegetables, grains, protein, and dairy. A meal should contain roughly half fruits and vegetables, and the other half grains and proteins, including items in the dairy food sub-group.

- Medical diet types have been developed to accommodate patients that are unable to eat certain foods due to allergies or physical inability. They include regular diet, soft diet, mechanical soft diet, puréed diet, liquid diet, and diabetic diet.
- There are many factors that can cause an individual to refuse or be unable to eat a nutritional diet including inability to chew, swallow, or digest, physical inability to feed, memory or cognitive impairment, and cultural restrictions.
- Body mechanics are the ways an individual carries or holds themselves, and range of motion is the movement capability of a body's specific joint.
- Practicing proper use of body mechanics and range of motion exercises will keep patients, family, and staff comfortable and safe during the various tasks performed in healthcare facilities.
- Body mechanics includes the way someone carries or holds their body, and a patient's position and posture dictate how their body is positioned when supporting or moving themselves.
  - Positions include supine (laying on back), prone (laying on stomach), and lateral (laying on side).
  - Postures include static (standing, sitting, laying), dynamic (moving), kyphosis (curved shoulders), and lordosis (spine curvature).
- Range of Motion (ROM) includes active ROM (completed by the patient), active assisted ROM (completed by the patient and CNA/HHA), and passive ROM (completed by the CNA/HHA).
  - Common ROM exercises include adduction, abduction, flexion, extension, pronation, supination, internal/external rotation, deviation, and opposition.
- During the aging process, body systems go through changes, and older people tend to lose some of the body functions once provided through the five senses.
- Older patients are at a higher risk for infections and falls.
- The most evident and noticeable changes for the aging person occur across the five senses: sight, hearing, taste, smell, and touch.

BASIC NURSING SKILLS

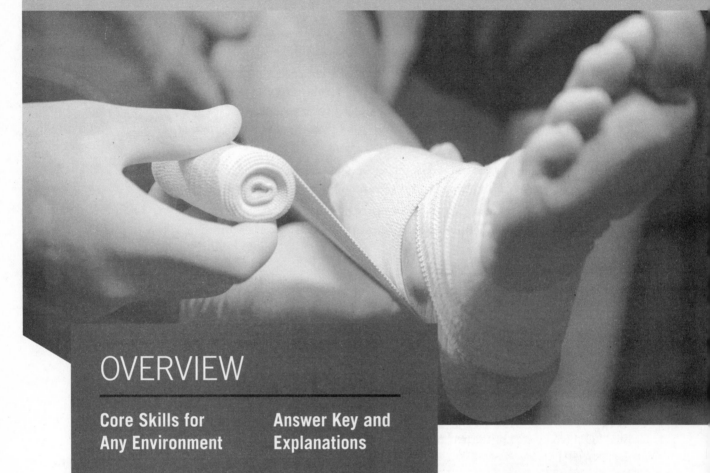

OVERVIEW

CORE SKILLS FOR ANY ENVIRONMENT

CNAs and HHAs can work in many different environments, including nursing homes, hospitals, rehabilitation centers, private homes, assisted living facilities, and more. No matter the location or circumstances surrounding their typical work requirements, many of a CNA's and HHA's duties revolve around core nursing skills that are outlined in this chapter. These skills include ones that are necessary to keep patients and staff healthy and safe.

INFECTION CONTROL

Infection prevention and control is one of the most important sets of protocols to follow for CNAs and HHAs. In medical facilities, patients bring many types of germs and illnesses that can easily spread into the facility to the employees and other patients. All staff should focus on controlling or preventing the possible spread, even when completing small tasks. Handwashing is a crucial part of infection control and the CNA and HHA exams.

Infections are caused by exposure to a pathogen. **Pathogens** are microorganisms that can cause illness and disease.

Bacteria are pathogens that can live both inside and outside of the human body. When they enter the body, they replicate quickly and can cause tissue damage in addition to infection. Hospital-acquired infections, or nosocomial infections, are caused by viral, fungal, and bacterial pathogens. Some of the most common types are bloodstream infection, pneumonia (often ventilator-associated pneumonia), urinary tract infection, and surgical site infection.

A **virus** is a type of pathogen that cannot thrive outside of the human body, but, once it enters, it infects other cells and is responsible for a wide range of infections. These infections include the common cold and flu.

Fungi are microorganisms that include yeasts and molds. Candidiasis is a fungal infection caused by a yeast called *Candida*. A common species of Candida that causes infection in people is *Candida albicans*. Though there are millions of different kinds of fungi, only around 300 of them are pathogenic. Pathogenic fungi are more likely to infect those with weakened immune systems. They can infect an individual in many ways, including direct skin contact, inhalation, and ingestion.

Protozoa love moisture and are often found in contaminated water, encapsulated in cysts, and in parasites, which means they need another organism to survive. Malaria is a red blood cell infection caused by protozoa.

Here are the pathogens mentioned above and the common infections they cause:

COMMON PATHOGENS	
PATHOGEN	**COMMON INFECTION**
Bacteria	*Salmonella, Staphylococcus,* and *E. coli*
Virus	the common cold, the flu, and COVID-19
Fungi	candidiasis, ringworm, nail infections
Protozoa	malaria, dysentery

The Chain of Infection

The Chain of Infection is made of six links and shows how infections begin and spread. Every link must be present for the infection to occur. In thinking of each component as a link, remember that a break in just one link will halt the spread of infection. Handwashing is the most efficient way to break the chain and stop infection.

This illustration shows the six links in The Chain of Infection:

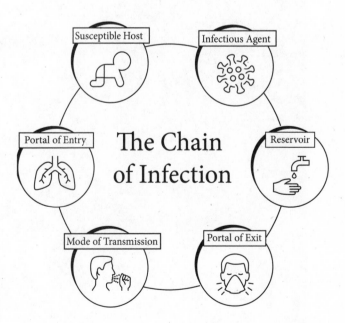

Infectious Agent—The germ that enters the bloodstream and causes infection. Not all germs cause infection. For example, we have germs on the outside of our skin that pose no problems. However, when a germ from your skin enters the bloodstream, an infection can occur.

Reservoir—The place where germs can live and multiply. Some germs thrive in heat, while others thrive in the cold. Reservoirs can be living organisms such as humans or animals, but they can also be objects and surfaces, such as doorknobs, counters, and bedrails.

Portal of Exit—An exit from the reservoir that allows the germ to spread. For example, if germs sit on a countertop and then someone touches the countertop, their hand becomes the portal of exit as it allows the germs to move to a new location. Other examples of portals of exit are feces, vomit, blood, and air.

Mode of Transmission—How the germ is spread. There are a variety of transmission modes, including direct contact (skin-to-skin, skin-to-object, skin-to-fluids etc.) and airborne transmission (coughing, sneezing, talking, etc.).

Portal of Entry—Movement of a germ from the reservoir to the host. The host is the person or other entity that now carries the germ. Open wounds, bodily fluids, eating or drinking, and breathing are all portals of entry. This is basically how the germ gets into the body.

Susceptible Host—Not every germ that enters the body will cause an infection because of our natural defense mechanisms called immunity. Therefore, the germ must have a susceptible host to continue growing and multiplying into a full-blown infection. A susceptible host is often a young person (such as an infant), an older person, or a person with a weakened immune system like those who have chronic illnesses, are stressed, or are fatigued.

Breaking the Chain of Infection

Infection control breaks at least one link in this chain. The most common way to break the chain is to practice proper and regular handwashing. We will cover the process of handwashing later in this chapter. For now, know that you break the infection chain in multiple locations when you practice proper handwashing techniques. The following are examples of how handwashing can break the infection chain:

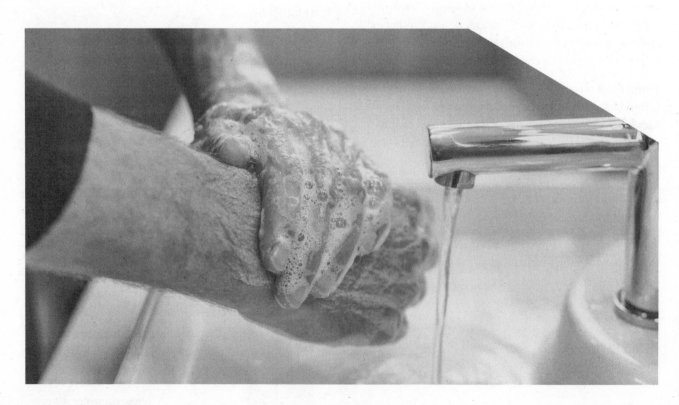

Reservoir—If a CNA or HHA has germs on their hands, their hands become the reservoir. Washing their hands breaks the chain because it kills the germs. Their hands are no longer a reservoir.

Portal of Exit—If a CNA or HHA touches a toilet seat and gets germs on their hands, they should wash their hands before touching the doorknob. Since the handwashing killed the germs, they were not successful in exiting and surviving.

Mode of Transportation—This is the most common way handwashing can stop the chain of infection. Hands are the number one most common mode of transportation as we touch all types of objects and surfaces throughout the day. In addition, during care, skin-to-skin contact is often required, and handwashing ensures that the hands are no longer a mode of transportation.

Portal of Entry—CNAs and HHAs encounter a multitude of surfaces with possible germs, including skin, medical tools, and various bodily fluids. Handwashing decreases the opportunity for the CNA to become a portal of entry.

Susceptible Host—CNA and HHA work is both physically and mentally taxing. Aides are the first point of contact for the patient and spend the most time with them providing daily care. To decrease the likelihood of becoming a susceptible host, CNAs and HHAs should wash their hands often so they do not pick up germs that can decrease their overall immune system. Get proper rest, eat a balanced diet, and use standard precautions to stay healthy.

Safety Precautions

Safety precautions are in place to ensure that patients and medical personnel resist possible infection. These precautions reduce the risk of infection by mandating

Universal Precautions

Safety practices introduced by CDC in the 1980s in response to the AIDS epidemic.

Guides medical personnel to assume all patients have the potential to be infectious through blood-borne pathogens; aides avoid contact with patient's bodily fluids.

Standard Precautions

CDC adjusts Universal Precautions to include more preventative measures.

Expands guidelines to include personal protective equipment (PPE), handwashing, disinfection, sterilization, vaccination, and monitoring of potential outbreaks.

Transmission-based Precautions

CDC offers guidelines for those suspected or confirmed to have an infectious illness.

These guidelines are in addition to and alongside Standard Precautions. They include guidance for precautions regarding contact, droplets, and airborne illnesses.

use of personal protective equipment (PPE) like gloves, goggles, and face shields, teaching proper and safe handling of all items that may contain a patient's bodily fluids, and requiring thorough disinfection and sterilization of surfaces and tools.

The terms Universal Precautions and Standard Precautions are currently used interchangeably in medical literature and instructions.

Standard Precautions

There are several components to standard precautions that work together to ensure the safety of both the patient and the provider from the spread of infection.

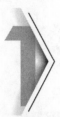 **Hand Hygiene**—This is the most critical part of infection control. You can fail the entire CNA or HHA exam if you do not wash your hands properly. More in-depth information will be discussed in the next section.

 **Personal Protective Equipment (PPE)**—This includes gloves, masks, gowns, and additional facial protection (goggles, shield, etc.). Each workplace must have the type of PPE required based on the type of precautions in place. For example, droplet precautions require a full gown, which is above and beyond Standard Precautions.

Respiratory Hygiene and Cough Etiquette—Covering your mouth and nose with the inside of your elbow helps to reduce the spread of droplets and airborne germs. In addition, there are guidelines for patient location (with others, isolated, etc.) based on the type of respiratory concerns they have.

 **Patient Equipment**—Cleaning patient equipment both before and after use is vital. Never assume a piece of equipment is clean. Standard precautions provide guidance on how to clean equipment and what type of cleaner to use to ensure that germs are killed.

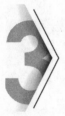

 **Environmental Cleaning and Linens**—Changing linens whenever soiled, and at least every other day when in an acute setting, can help to increase the cleanliness and health of the patient overall. In addition, the room itself should be frequently cleaned throughout the day to reduce the opportunity for reservoirs to accumulate, thus restricting germ growth and spread.

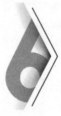 **Sharps Safety**—Although you will most likely not be directly administering injections, you may assist others in doing so. Sharps can carry infectious pathogens and need to be disposed of in a specific sharps container. If you are at a patient's home, a sharps container should be on-site as it is required with the delivery of any needle-based treatments.

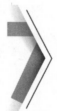 **Waste Disposal**—There are two main types of waste: common garbage and clinical waste. Common garbage items include food containers, paper, and old food. Clinical waste, which is considered contaminated and possibly infectious, is any waste that possibly has bodily fluids, secretions, or blood on it. Clinical waste must be disposed of in a specific manner and separately from common waste to avoid any possible spread of infection. Treat clinical waste carefully and dispose of it following the guidelines outlined by your workplace.

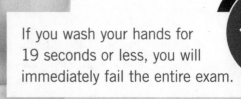

If you wash your hands for 19 seconds or less, you will immediately fail the entire exam.

Handwashing

Handwashing is so important not only in infection control but on the CNA and HHA exam as well. The first part of your skills test for the CNA and HHA exam will be handwashing, regardless of what other care skills are selected for you to complete. Your handwashing will be timed, and the proctor is dedicated to the stopwatch. The handwashing requirement is 20 seconds.

The following are detailed instructions on best practices for washing your hands. Make sure to practice this skill daily, timing yourself to ensure you reach at least 20 seconds before rinsing. There is no penalty for washing them too long.

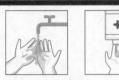

STEP 1:
Wet your hands with clean, warm, running water and apply soap.

STEP 2:
Away from the water, lather your hands by rubbing them with the soap, creating bubbles or foam. Make sure to rub the front and back of your hands, including your nails and rings. A common mistake is to rub your hands under the water. Do not do that. This does not actually clean your hands.

STEP 3:
Scrub your hands for at least 20 seconds. This includes lathering your wrists, hands, and fingers and cleaning your fingernails by rubbing them against the palm of your other hand while keeping your hands and fingers pointed down toward the sink. This will ensure that both your hands are clean and you have passed the time limit of this section of the exam.

STEP 4:
Rinse your hands well under the clean, running water while keeping your hands and fingers pointed down toward the sink. Do not use standing water, such as a bowl of water or water held in a sink.

STEP 5:
Dry your hands with a clean, dry towel (linen or disposable) and make sure to dry all hand and wrist surfaces. Use another clean, dry towel or a knee/foot control to turn off the water. Dispose of the towel(s) in the proper waste receptacle. Do not wipe your hands on your pants or shirt to dry them, and make sure not to touch the inside of the sink at any time while handwashing.

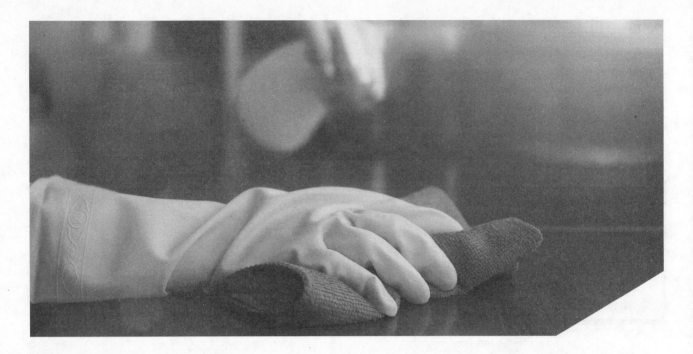

Disinfection and Sterilization

CNAs and HHAs should always adhere to proper sterilization and disinfection to prevent the spread of illness or disease. On top of this, aides should properly handle contaminated items to reduce the contact between the items and themselves or anything in their surroundings.

Sterilization

Sterilization means subjecting an item to high heat, often in the form of steam, to kill all microorganisms on the item. The materials that medical instruments are made of can withstand the heat from the process of sterilizing. Generally, this material is metal, but there are some plastic-based instruments that can handle a lower heat that is still effective in sterilizing. These lower heat sterilizations involve gasses, such as ethylene oxide, instead of steam. Hand tools used in a surgery are perfect examples of instruments that need sterilization. They are metal instruments that can be properly sterilized before and after surgery.

Disinfection

Disinfection means using a chemical compound to kill the microorganisms on a surface. However, disinfectants (the chemical compounds used to disinfect) do not kill all microorganisms like sterilization does.

Disinfectants are made of different types of chemicals and have their own applications and mixing ratios. Aides should follow all labels on the chemicals when mixing and using a disinfectant. Common disinfectants include alcohols, chlorine or chlorine-based products, formaldehyde, and hydrogen peroxide.

Proper Handling and Disposal

When handling items that could be contaminated, wear personal protective equipment (PPE) and hold the items away from your body. This will help to reduce the risk of self-contamination. A good example of this is handling dirty linens. When doing so, wear gloves, and hold the linens as far away from your body as possible. This will help reduce the spread of fluids and other contaminants present on the linens. Do not hold the linens against yourself, even if it is easier to do so.

If a piece of equipment, tool, or other object is used and meant to be thrown away after, you should correctly handle disposal following your workplace guidelines for clinical waste. Any bodily fluid or chemical-covered waste must be disposed of in a container that is meant for clinical waste. Clinical waste cannot be mixed with general waste because general waste is not handled with enough safety to keep the harmful microorganisms and chemicals contained.

MINI-QUIZ: INFECTION CONTROL

> **Directions:** Read each question below and choose the correct answer from the four choices provided. Only one choice is correct, so choose carefully.

1. The second step in the hand-washing process is
   - **A.** rinsing your hands.
   - **B.** scrubbing your hands.
   - **C.** turning on the water.
   - **D.** lathering your hands.

2. How many links are in the chain of infection?
   - **A.** 4
   - **B.** 5
   - **C.** 6
   - **D.** 8

3. The single most effective way to break the chain of infection is to
   - **A.** wash your hands.
   - **B.** cover your cough.
   - **C.** disinfect the counters.
   - **D.** stay home when sick.

4. The link in the chain of infection that has to do with how the germ is spread from one person to another is called the
   - **A.** portal of exit.
   - **B.** mode of transmission.
   - **C.** portal of entry.
   - **D.** infectious agent.

5. Transmission-based precautions require _____ in comparison to universal precautions.
   - **A.** more PPE
   - **B.** less PPE
   - **C.** the same PPE
   - **D.** different PPE

6. Which of the following is an example of a protozoa germ?
   - **A.** The flu
   - **B.** Chicken pox
   - **C.** Malaria
   - **D.** Common cold

7. Which of the following cleaning processes are done to a room throughout the day?
   - **A.** Disinfection
   - **B.** Sterilization
   - **C.** Sanitation
   - **D.** Decontamination

8. How many links of the chain of infection need to be broken to stop the spread of infection?
   - **A.** 2
   - **B.** 4
   - **C.** 6
   - **D.** 1

9. How many seconds minimum should you wash your hands before rinsing them?
   - **A.** 10 seconds
   - **B.** 20 seconds
   - **C.** 30 seconds
   - **D.** 60 seconds

10. The process by which medical instruments are subjected to intense heat to kill all microorganisms is called
    - **A.** disinfection.
    - **B.** sterilization.
    - **C.** sanitation.
    - **D.** decontamination.

ANSWER KEY AND EXPLANATIONS

1. D	3. A	5. A	7. A	9. B
2. C	4. B	6. C	8. D	10. B

1. **The correct answer is D.** The second step in the handwashing process is lathering your hands. This occurs after turning on the water (choice C) and wetting your hands but before scrubbing (choice B) and rinsing (choice A) your hands.

2. **The correct answer is C.** There are six links in the chain of infection—Infectious Agent, Reservoir, Portal of Exit, Mode of Transmission, Portal of Entry, and Susceptible Host. All other answers are incorrect.

3. **The correct answer is A.** The single most effective way to break the chain of infection is to sever one link. Handwashing can stop all six links. Covering your cough (choice B), disinfecting the counters (choice C), and staying home when you are sick (choice D) are all helpful but not as helpful as washing your hands.

4. **The correct answer is B.** The mode of transmission is the "how" link—it tells you how the germ is transferred from the reservoir to the host. The portal of exit (choice A) is how the disease left the reservoir. The portal of entry (choice C) is how the germ entered into the body. The infectious agent (choice D) is the germ itself.

5. **The correct answer is A.** Transmission-based precautions require both PPE outlined in the Universal Precautions and additional PPE such as gowns and face shields. Choices B, C, and D are incorrect.

6. **The correct answer is C.** Malaria is an example of a protozoa germ. The flu (choice A), chicken pox (choice B), and the common cold (choice D) are all examples of a virus.

7. **The correct answer is A.** Disinfection is the process of cleaning and killing most germs quickly as different cares and activities are completed. Sterilization (choice B) requires extreme heat to kill all the germs and cannot be completed throughout the day. Sanitation (choice C) and decontamination (choice D) do not include cleaning throughout a day either.

8. **The correct answer is D.** Only one link in the chain of infection needs to be broken to stop the spread of infection, as all six links must be completed to spread from the reservoir to the host. Choices A, B, and C are incorrect.

9. **The correct answer is B.** To ensure proper cleaning and to pass the CNA and HHA skills test for hand hygiene, you should wash your hands for a minimum of 20 seconds. If you wash your hands for 10 seconds (choice A), you will fail the exam. If you wash your hands for 30 seconds (choice C) or 60 seconds (choice D), you may not be penalized, but washing for these lengths of time is not necessary.

10. **The correct answer is B.** Sterilization is the process of killing all microorganisms. Disinfection (choice A) does not kill all germs but most of them. Sanitation (choice C) is the process of hygienically removing waste. Decontamination (choice D) is not applicable to the cleaning of medical instruments because it is used during a contaminated and unsafe environment, such as an oil spill.

SAFETY

Having safety protocols to follow not only helps to prevent accidents, but also aids in dealing with an accident in an efficient and timely way. Safety measures can be prescribed for accidents as small as a burn from a hot cup of coffee to accidents as big as preventing a pathogen from spreading. As a CNA or HHA, it is important to be prepared for any emergencies that may occur when caring for a patient and to be aware of the facility's procedures for responding to an emergency. Since emergency response teams can take time to respond, it is also important to know basic first aid to be able to provide care to a patient during an emergency, including if the patient collapses, chokes, or stops breathing. There are also precautions that a CNA or HHA can take to prevent safety issues, including taking steps to avoid falls and to help unstable or wandering patients. Lastly, the Occupational Safety and Health Administration (OSHA) provides information to all workplaces about how to maintain safety standards, and CNAs and HHAs should pay particular attention to their guidelines for preventing infections via bloodborne pathogens.

Emergency Preparedness

Every workplace has an **emergency preparedness** training that you will complete. However, it can be overwhelming in the moment to remember what exactly is required of you when in a large medical building such as a hospital or a nursing home. Unlike a traditional evacuation response to fires and other emergencies, these facilities are designed for those inside to **shelter in place** in an emergency. In the case of a fire, fireproof doors will automatically close when the alarm sounds. This traps the fire to one location of the building and can also help with damages from hurricanes and tornadoes. Residents and

The term *stat* is used when there is an emergency or critical situation within a hospital, and something must be done at once. For example: "Remove the patients closest to the fire stat!"

staff will stay in their rooms with the door closed unless directed by emergency personnel to evacuate. If evacuation is ordered, the ambulatory patients are directed to join hands and are evacuated first. Bedridden patients can either be transferred to a wheelchair if there is time to do so, or they can be transferred onto a blanket and pulled to the exit if necessary.

If you are near the fire, you may be asked to use the **RACE** method, which stands for Remove/Rescue, Activate/Alarm, Contain/Confine, Extinguish/Evacuate. The first step is to remove everyone from danger, including patients, staff, and visitors, by moving them away from the fire. Next, alert emergency services by pulling a fire alarm, calling 911, or contacting responders in the building. Then, try to contain or confine the

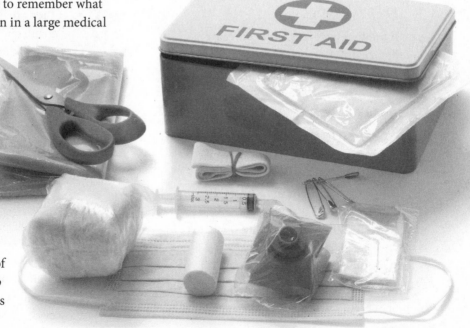

fire by closing doors and windows. If it's a small fire, you may try to extinguish it, or wait for instructions from emergency services to begin evacuating the building. Hospitals have individual evacuation plans for their specific facility. The first to be evacuated are the patients closest to the hazard.

First Aid

First aid is the immediate and temporary care given to an individual until skilled medical care can be given. Being able to apply basic first aid to a patient in an accident or emergency is an extremely important skill that all nursing assistants should possess, as it can mean life or death for a patient in extreme situations. The basic steps of applying first aid in an emergency are as follows:

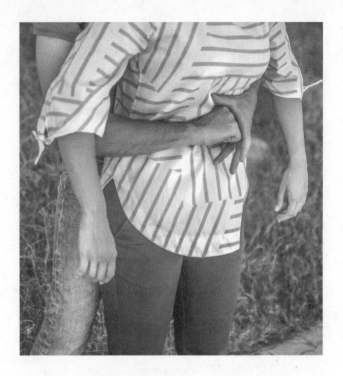

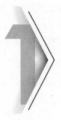

Assess the situation before administering care. Rushing into a scene without first checking the surroundings could lead to further injury, especially if there is an environmental hazard. Assessing the situation will help you gather information on the individual's needs.

Check for responsiveness and call for help.

- **If another person is with you:** Have them call 911 or another appropriate emergency number and have them attain an AED if available.

- **If you are alone:** You will have to call for help while checking the individual as effectively as you can.

- **If the individual is responsive:** Ask for consent to assess and assist them. Be sure to wear any PPE that is available for you. Ask the individual if they know what is wrong with them and what happened. Assess them head-to-toe.

- **If the individual appears unresponsive:** Shout to try to get a response from them, tap their shoulder (or bottom of their feet if they are an infant), and check for breathing. Only check to see if they are responsive for 5-10 seconds before acting.

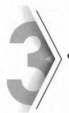

Provide first aid based on your assessment.

- **If they are breathing:** Treat the individual with any necessary first aid that you have the knowledge and training to do. If they do not require immediate first aid, then they can be rolled onto their side in a recovery position. Do not move an individual if information gathered hints at them having an injury that can be worsened by movement (such as a spinal injury or head trauma).

- **If they are not breathing:** Position the individual face up on a flat, solid surface. From there, begin CPR until the individual's condition improves and they are conscious and breathing, until an AED is provided or until Emergency Medical Services (EMS) arrive.

ADULT	INFANT
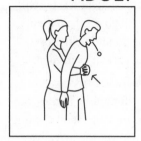	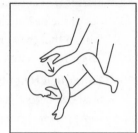

Choking

If you suspect that a patient is choking, before taking any action, you must **ask them if they are choking.** Any coughing, gasps for air, or speaking indicates they are not choking. If they can make noises or cough, use calm words to help them relax. Encourage them to breathe through their nose to reduce the struggle. As they start to calm down, you can also offer them some cold water to help the food go down. If the patient isn't making any sounds or coughing, attempt to expel the lodged object using the Heimlich maneuver.

Heimlich Maneuver and Abdominal Thrusts

Before attempting the **Heimlich Maneuver**, have the patient stand up, if possible, as it works best in this position. Use thrusts to the abdomen to dislodge blockages in the airway that are causing an individual to choke. To properly execute the thrusts, make a fist in one hand, place the thumb side of that fist on the abdomen, place the other hand over the fist, and thrust inward and upward. This will push air from the lungs out and will expel the blockage. If an infant is choking, abdominal thrusts are not used because they could cause harm to the infant. To try to clear an infant's airway, place them face down over your forearm and then give five strong back slaps between their shoulder blades.

Safety Practices during Activities of Daily Living (ADLs)

When caring for a patient during Activities of Daily Living (ADLs), there is always potential for safety concerns to arise, and it is the CNA's or HHA's responsibility to prevent or respond to any safety issues. For example, part of ADLs involves moving and transferring patients, which can result in falls if not properly completed. If there is a question about safety hazards, ask the supervisor about the hazard or situation and **alert** others of any dangers. When you alert someone of a danger, provide a clear message about the danger to avoid confusion. The following are common best practices to help increase patients' safety.

Falls

It is impossible to account for all possible reasons that a patient may fall. However, there are common struggles and situations that increase the risk. The following are common reasons falls happen:

- **Age and Fragility**—As age increases, so does the likelihood of falls. As people age, their bodies become more fragile, and they are less able to lift their feet as high when walking and transitioning between surfaces like wood and carpet. In addition, some patients, regardless of age, have fragile bodies that are more prone to falls due to weak bones or joints.

- **Vision Quality**—Decreased vision increases risk for falls. When someone cannot see well, obstacles are not as obvious.

- **Poor Balance and Coordination**—Some illnesses and medications have a substantial effect on balance and coordination. Vertigo (dizziness) and poor coordination due to muscle weakness or tremors can both increase fall risk.

- **Unsafe Flooring Transitions**—Because walking may become difficult as a person ages, it is important for flooring to be safe and secure. Facilities should repair flooring that has untacked carpet or loose rugs and provide proper signage for wet floors to prevent falls.

- **Clutter**—This can be both controlled (due to patient belongings) or beyond their control (like walkers in the hallway). Nursing aides should work with the patient and facility to clear clutter and remove unnecessary obstacles.

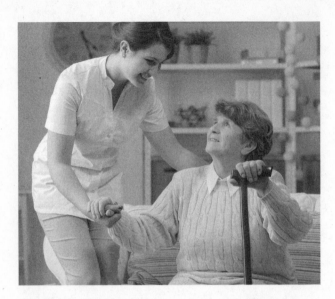

Ways to Prevent Falls

Although there are concrete ways to prevent falls, the most important and valuable resource a CNA and HHA has is an understanding of a patient's physical, emotional, and cognitive skills. Being aware of these factors can help a nursing aide care for a patient in a way that prevents falls. In addition, knowing the environment in which the patient resides is also extremely important. Daily inspection of both the patient for any changes to their physical, emotional, and cognitive abilities and the patient's environment for any hazards will help keep the patient safe.

Tools and Procedures

As a person progresses in their illness, they will naturally lose physical and cognitive skills. This can result in necessary changes to care to prevent falls. CNAs and HHAs should be aware of the procedures and tools available to help prevent patient falls. Here are examples of safety precautions for preventing falls:

Bedrails are restraints and may never be used to prevent falls from a bed without a doctor's order.

- **Bed and Chair Alarms**—These are simple alarms that alert staff when a patient has gotten out of the bed or chair. It will go off if a patient falls so that the aide can respond quickly to assess injuries and help the patient as needed.

- **Lower Bed Heights**—If a patient is using a hospital bed (as is the case for all nursing homes and some private homes) there is an adjustable height option. This can be used to lower the bed closer to the floor to prevent injuries if a fall does occur.

- **Use a Floor Mat**—This absorbent mat can be placed parallel to the bed to soften a fall should the patient fall out of bed.

- **Encourage the Use of Aids**—This includes bedrails, railings in the hallway and bathroom, prescribed canes/walkers, and transfer assistance. Eyeglasses should always be kept within the reach of the patient to improve vision quality and prevent potential falls. These aids can be used during transfers and when walking, which are common times for falls to occur.

- **Wear Proper Shoes or Nonslip Socks**—Some patients use wheelchairs or walk infrequently, which may make shoes or nonslip socks seem unnecessary. However, wearing proper shoes or nonslip socks allows for safer transfers from the bed to the wheelchair and for walking, even if it is only minimal steps to a commode or bathing chair.

- **Complete Range of Motion/Exercise**—Patients are prescribed specific daily range of motion exercises to help maintain strength and flexibility. It is important to encourage these to help prevent falls through strength in muscle tone and flexibility. Stiff joints and decreased strength directly affect falls.

- **Document Daily Observations**—Never underestimate the power of personal observations. A CNA or HHA spends the most amount of time with a patient when compared with any other staff. They may notice physical or cognitive changes before they are officially documented. Report these observations to the nurse and take extra safety precautions to prevent falls.

Using Bedrails

Bedrails are present on all hospital beds. Most beds have four rails: two on either side, one at the head of the bed, and one at the foot of the bed. The use of bedrails is a form of restraint, which can sometimes further endanger a patient. Restrained patients can develop muscle weakness, cognitive or behavioral changes, and physical injuries. A patient restrained with bedrails may become seriously injured if they try to climb over the bedrails, or they may develop feelings of isolation. A patient may also become wedged in a bedrail or wedged between the bedrail and the mattress, which is called **entrapment**. Catheters should never be taped to a bedrail because the catheter should be lower than the patient's bladder. Taping it to the bedrail can cause a backflow of urine, which leads to infection.

However, if used properly and with careful observation, there are some benefits to using one or more of the four rails. A **head-based bedrail** can be engaged to help with transferring out of the bed, repositioning within the bed, and stabilizing after standing up. Encourage the use of this bedrail for ambulatory and mobile patients. This type of use is not a restraint. If a patient is permanently bedridden, the bedrails should always be raised to guard them. This, however, is a restraint and requires a doctor's order along with frequent checks to ensure safety of the resident.

Proper Wheelchair Use

Many patients will need assistance with mobility and will need the use of a wheelchair to get around. If the wheelchair is not used properly, a patient could become injured if they experience a fall or collide with something. When a patient is entering or leaving a wheelchair, lock the wheels and lift the footrests first. When transporting a patient in a wheelchair through an open door, check for traffic before going through to avoid collision. If a patient cannot climb into or out of a wheelchair on their own, use a transfer belt or lift. If a patient is anxious while being moved during a fire alarm or similar emergency, do not stop. Instead, calm them down by talking to them in a calm voice while still moving them to a safe location. Going down a wheelchair ramp backwards is the safest and most controlled method of doing so.

Helping Wandering Patients

Patients in a long-term care facility will often wander. If the patients are wandering in restricted or dangerous areas, they may need redirection. In addition, alarms may be in place to promote safety. The following are useful strategies to assist wandering patients:

- **Verbal Redirection**—When attempting to redirect a wandering resident, use the phrase, "It's so nice to walk with you." It is nonconfrontational and wandering patients can often be easily redirected simply by walking them back to the unit.

- **Tracking Bracelets**—These are simple bracelets that correlate with boundaries within the unit. When a resident goes beyond the boundary or attempts to go out the door, an alarm will sound, and the door may lock. This alerts staff that someone has gone too far.

- **Bed and Wheelchair Alarms**—These can be used for patients to alert staff when a patient with mobility issues has wandered away from their last location. Although this can be for falls as well, it is also a valuable tool for wandering patients.

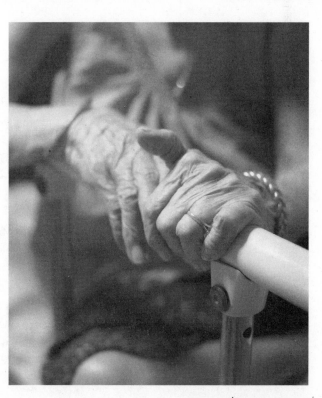

Occupational Safety and Health Administration (OSHA)

The Occupational Safety and Health Administration (OSHA) is the federal agency that oversees setting and enforcing standard regulations in the workplace. These regulations are applicable to all workplaces in the US. Individual companies will also have their own regulations that are based on or are separate from the regulations set by OSHA. Either way, these regulations are meant to prevent injury, violence, and harassment for employees, patrons, and patients.

CNAs or HHAs that feel in danger or uncomfortable about a situation while at work should notify the proper individuals. For example, if an assault or threat of assault was directed toward someone at work, then the supervisor on duty should be notified. Assault, or even just the threat of assault, is workplace violence and is not tolerated. The supervisor on duty will have the knowledge and authority to act in solving this problem. It is important for all CNAs and HHAs to understand their rights to safety as employees in addition to their roles as care providers to patients. If an uncomfortable or dangerous situation arises in a home setting, inform

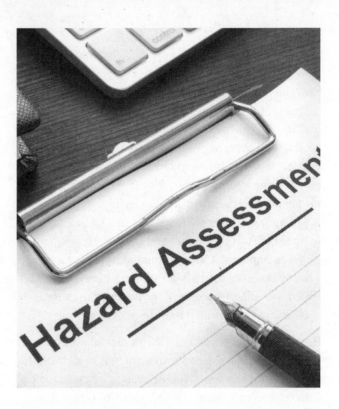

the nurse in charge of the matter. In this setting, the nurse takes the role of supervisor for the assistant and can help mediate the situation.

OSHA & Blood-borne Pathogens

In addition to workplace regulations regarding employee treatment, OSHA also dictates the planning, prevention, and disposal of **blood-borne pathogens.** The following list includes an overview of this regulation and what is expected from your workplace:

PLAN	PREPARE	TREAT
Every facility must have a plan in place for protecting the employees from blood-borne pathogens. This includes universal/standard precautions, PPE, and protocols for cares and sharp objects.	Every facility must also instruct its staff in how to prevent contact to reduce the spread of these pathogens and how to respond should contact occur. This also includes providing free vaccinations along with engineering controls like sharps containers.	Every facility must also provide free and comprehensive care for any employee that is exposed to blood-borne pathogens. This includes testing, treatment if found to be infected, and ongoing care related to exposure.

MINI-QUIZ: SAFETY

Directions: Read each question below and choose the correct answer from the four choices provided. Only one choice is correct, so choose carefully.

1. A safety precaution is
   A. the decision of the charge nurse.
   B. a personal choice.
   C. the choice of each facility.
   D. a national standard.

2. When is the most common time for a fall to occur?
   A. Mealtime
   B. While sleeping
   C. Bathtime
   D. During transfers

3. Glasses should always be kept
   A. in a case at the nurse's station.
   B. within the reach of the patient.
   C. alongside the patient's medications.
   D. around a patient's neck.

4. Why are bed and chair alarms useful for wandering patients?
   A. They notify family members when a patient has left the room/chair.
   B. They notify staff when a patient falls asleep.
   C. They notify the patient when they are about to fall.
   D. They notify staff when a patient is no longer in the bed or chair safely.

5. If a patient appears to be choking but can still cough, you should
   A. encourage them to breathe through their nose.
   B. hit their back.
   C. give the Heimlich Maneuver.
   D. blow in their face.

6. When should evacuation begin during a fire at a nursing home?
   A. As soon as the fire alarm goes off
   B. When the fire department arrives
   C. When smoke is visible
   D. When directed to by the assigned emergency point person

7. It is important for all patients to wear proper shoes or nonslip socks because doing so
   A. keeps their feet dry.
   B. prevents cracks in their heels.
   C. helps to prevent falls.
   D. boosts their self-esteem.

8. When transferring from the bed to a wheelchair, what is the most important step?
   A. Maneuvering the wheelchair close to the patient
   B. Putting on a gait belt before transferring
   C. Locking the wheels and lifting the footrests
   D. Putting nonstick socks or shoes on the patient

9. When moving a resident in a wheelchair, you should always
   A. go backwards down a ramp.
   B. keep the foot pedals up unless requested.
   C. go backwards around a corner.
   D. leave the gait belt on for ease of transfer.

10. Whose responsibility is it to prevent falls?
    A. The nurse
    B. The CNA
    C. The doctor
    D. All staff

ANSWER KEY AND EXPLANATIONS

1. D	**3.** B	**5.** A	**7.** C	**9.** A
2. D	**4.** D	**6.** D	**8.** C	**10.** D

1. **The correct answer is D.** There are standards in place on a national level concerning patient safety. The decision of the charge nurse (choice A), your personal choice (choice B), and the choice of each facility (choice C) cannot override an official safety precaution.

2. **The correct answer is D.** The most common time for a fall to occur is during transfers because a person is going from one surface to another. Often these surfaces are at different levels (such as a bed and a wheelchair) which increases the likelihood of a fall. During meals (choice A) a person is sitting down, making a fall unlikely. During sleep (choice B) is the second most common time for falls as patients may roll out of bed. Falls occurring during bathing (choice C) are low in number as a patient is sitting on a bathing chair. However, transfers that happen before and after the actual bathing are common times.

3. **The correct answer is B.** Glasses are considered a prescribed aid and not having them can increase the risk of falls. They should always be within reach of the resident. They should never be kept in a case by the nurse's station (choice A) or alongside the patient's medications (choice C) as that does not benefit the patient, and they should never have to ask to use them. They should never be kept around a patient's neck (choice D) as this can cause a choking hazard when in bed or during times of sleep, and they should be removed when the patient is in their bed.

4. **The correct answer is D.** Bed and chair alarms notify staff when a patient is no longer safely in their bed or chair. This may be due to a fall, the patient attempting to get up (possibly unsafely), or a patient shifting into an unsafe, near-falling position. Bed and chair alarms do not notify family (choice A); they are not useful in notifying staff of a patient's sleep patterns (choice B); and they are

not able to notify staff when a patient is about to fall (choice C) as they go off after the patient has left the bed or chair.

5. **The correct answer is A.** If a patient can still cough, they are not choking, but they are clearly having difficulty in some capacity. Breathing through their nose can help them calm down, which will open their throat more easily. Hitting their back (choice B) and blowing in their face (choice D) will offer no actual assistance. Giving the Heimlich Maneuver (choice C) will not help and can complicate the situation when the person is not truly choking.

6. **The correct answer is D.** In a nursing home, evacuation is not automatic as the facility is under a "shelter in place" directive because of the way it was built. Many times, evacuation is not necessary for all sections, and the compromised health of the residents can complicate matters if the staff attempts an evacuation. In every facility, there is an emergency point person (usually the administrator) that will be guided by the fire department about the evacuation. Choices A, B, and C are all incorrect.

7. **The correct answer is C.** Wearing proper shoes or nonslip socks is important to help prevent falls. When a patient is barefoot or wearing regular socks, they are more prone to slipping or tripping. Keeping their feet dry (choice A) and preventing cracks in their heels (choice B) are both possible added benefits but not the main reason for requiring them. Also, boosting their self-esteem (choice D) is a possible benefit as it may provide a complete look for the patient (especially in a long-term care facility), but safety is the number one priority.

8. **The correct answer is C.** Locking the wheels and lifting the footrests is the most important step as it ensures the wheelchair is stable before the transfer.

Choices A, B, and D are all useful, but they are not more important.

9. **The correct answer is A.** Going backwards down a ramp is the safest option as it decreases the likelihood of the patient falling out as they are at an angle. You should always put the foot pedals down (choice B). You should never go backwards around a corner (choice C) or leave the gait belt on (choice D) as both are considered unsafe.

10. **The correct answer is D.** The responsibility to prevent falls should be shared by all staff. This starts with the CNA (choice B) who interacts with the patient multiple times a day. The nurse (choice A) who sees the patient several times a day and receives reports from the CNA and the doctor (choice C), who may see the patient only once a day or once a week and receive reports from the nurse, are also responsible for preventing falls.

NOTES

DATA COLLECTION AND VITAL SIGNS

CNAs and HHAs are responsible for **collecting data** on patients and checking their **vital signs** throughout each day. The information gathered through collecting data and checking vital signs can help with patient diagnosis and treatment, so these skills are an essential part of being a health aide. Gathering patient data involves administering questionnaires that ask questions about their health condition and background, running assessments on a patient to uncover needs, and observing the patient for any changes to their health. Vital signs include important information about the body like temperature, blood pressure, and pulse. A CNA or HHA should know how to check these vital signs and record what they find. In addition, they should know when to report any troubling readings to the nurse or doctor. Understanding and monitoring a patient's health through data and vital signs helps to create a care plan that can best serve each patient's unique needs.

Data Collection

Data collection is used both when a patient is admitted to a medical unit and during their treatment and care. It is the duty of health professionals to keep a patient's information (both personal and medical) **confidential**. This means that it is private between the medical personnel and the patient.

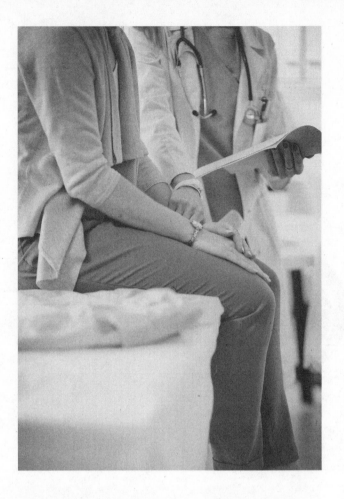

When a medical professional first evaluates a patient, they gather data by interviewing the patient or having them fill out a questionnaire. Questionnaires provide **quantitative data**, numbers and figures that can help create a full picture of the patient's needs. For example, a new patient may be asked how many medications they take daily and in what quantities. This information gives insight into what treatments they currently receive and what might be the best way to move forward with treatment. If a resident or patient is unable to provide answers to these questions, data collection may need to include a family member or other trusted person. Sometimes, when there is not another person available, data collection will require the health professional to research through previous records to gather all necessary and related information.

Another type of quantitative data that CNAs and HHAs collect are a patient's **intake and output (I&O)**. I&O is the balance between the fluids that a patient takes in and the fluids that they excrete. A patient should have equal input and output. If a patient excretes more than they take in, they could become dehydrated. If they take in more than they excrete, they could retain excess fluid. Check the patient's care plan for an I&O chart that can help with making these calculations and report any severe changes to the nurse.

Data can also be collected by running assessments or tests on a patient. This is **qualitative data collection** because the assessment or test is done for more specific findings than the broad range of questions on a questionnaire. For example, a sleep study is used to test if the patient experiences sleep apnea, but a questionnaire on sleeping problems can identify many different sleep complications that do not show up on the physical test, such as quality of sleep.

Testing, Observing, and Monitoring

Testing for detection is a part of the process of diagnosing a patient. There are many different tests that can be done for either a singular condition or multiple conditions. **Lab tests**, for example, can be done on samples from a patient to determine the presence of infection. Lab tests can also be used for monitoring, such as verifying whether the treatment is working. Tests can also be done in the office or patient's room, but they are not the same types of tests that are done in a lab.

Here are examples of some of the kinds of tests and where they are typically completed:

EXAMPLES OF TYPES OF TESTS	
USUALLY COMPLETED IN PATIENT'S ROOM OR AT THE LONG-TERM CARE FACILITY	**USUALLY COMPLETED IN A HOSPITAL/LAB**
Cognitive tests: measure skills involving learning and problem-solving.	**Guaiac tests**: check for hidden blood in a patient's stool.
Urine tests: look for hidden proteins, ketones, and sugar in a patient's urine.	**Biopsy**: used to detect cancer.
Blood tests: can detect sugar, ketones, and cholesterol in a patient's blood. Can also be used to detect diabetes.	**CT scan**: also called a CAT scan. Series of x-ray images compiled together to look for problems internally.
Spirometry tests: measure how effectively the lungs work.	**Tympanometry**: measures the movement of the eardrum with response to air pressure.
Neurological exam: Check for response of dilation, tracking, and reflexes.	**MRI**: Magnetic Resonance Imaging is used in radiology to create a scan of the inside of your body, especially organs. More sensitive than a CT scan.
Range of motion test: Determines how far a resident can bend, flex, stand, walk, etc.	**Electrocardiogram (ECG)**: measures how well the heart works by recording its electrical signals.

In addition to the above tests, patients are also observed and monitored. Though it is not specifically a test, **observation** is extremely important for the assessment and monitoring of a patient, and all five senses and active listening skills should be used to observe them. CNAs or HHAs should notice any changes in the patient's appearance, vital signs, odor, or ability to respond. The CNA should also listen to any statements made by the patient about how they are feeling, as these statements can sometimes point to underlying issues. The CNA or HHA should report any changes that they observe, and flow charts are often used in patient charts to assess the changes in a patient from one period to another. When reporting observations, make sure to use clear language and to be objective—report only what you observed, not your opinions.

If you observe serious injuries or changes, like complications after a fall or drastic changes to weight or blood pressure, report those to the nurse immediately. Document these changes in the patient's chart and follow the nurse's instructions about how to proceed. Also, if the patient reports any allegations of abuse, these statements need to be immediately reported to the nurse. All other statements that point to a patient's health and well-being should be documented in their chart or, if requested by the resident, they can be reported to the Long-Term Care Ombudsman, an elected official representing patient concerns.

Assessing a patient is not only a part of testing but also important for **monitoring**, which is utilizing tests, assessment, and observation to see if a patient's condition is improving or declining. Monitoring is constantly happening every day that the patient is under the care of professionals. Even if it is only via observations, they are still being monitored for the most basic of status updates. Monitoring is not, however, only for passive observations at varying times by the CNA. Monitoring can also be used for detecting changes in a patient throughout the course of seconds, minutes, and hours.

Often this monitoring is assisted with a device that is actively testing a vital sign of a patient to detect any changes. A good example of one of these devices is the **doppler device**, which is a hand-held monitor that detects blood flow, blood pressure, and heartbeats. Another good example is the **oximeter**, which is a device that is placed over the nailbed of the finger to check oxygen saturation in the blood. If a patient has fingernail polish on their nails, it can disrupt the reading, so be sure to remove it if you receive a low reading on a patient wearing polish.

Temperature

Temperature in a human body is an important component to being healthy. The normal temperature range is

A temperature can be heavily affected by external variables. Some common ones are a dirty probe (make sure to clean before and after every use), drinking or eating cold foods (make sure to wait 15 minutes before rechecking an oral temperature), excessive sweat (wipe with a dry towel and check again), and a cold patient (warm them up and check again in 15 minutes).

97°-99° Fahrenheit for adults and 97°-100.3° Fahrenheit for infants. A temperature that is higher than normal is a **fever**, and it is often a condition brought on from an illness. Temperatures above 103°F are considered dangerous for adults, and an infant with a temperature above 100.4°F has a fever and should receive medical attention. If body temperature drops below 95°F, a patient is experiencing **hypothermia**.

Measuring temperature can be done in several ways, each with their own differing accuracies:

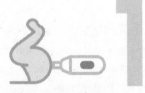

RECTAL TEMPERATURE:
Temperature is measured by inserting a thermometer into the rectum. This is the most accurate way to measure temperature but is almost always restricted to infants.

TEMPORAL TEMPERATURE:
Measuring temperature by using a temperature scanner that begins on the forehead and ends behind the ear. This is the second most accurate temperature reading after rectal temperature as it is measuring temperature via the temporal artery.

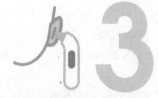

TYMPANIC TEMPERATURE:
This measurement is done by inserting a thermometer into the ear. This form of measuring temperature is not as accurate as taking rectal temperature, but it is more accurate than the following methods.

Vital Signs for the Heart and Lungs

Checking **vital signs** is an important process when monitoring patients and their condition. **Blood pressure** and **pulse** are the main vitals regarding blood and the heart. **Respiratory rate** and **oxygen saturation** are the main vitals for breathing and the lungs. Accurately recording these vitals is important, and they can tell you a lot about what a patient's body is doing.

Blood Pressure

Blood pressure refers to the pressure applied to the artery walls. There are two different types of blood pressure, and they are categorized based on what the ventricles do when there is pressure on the artery walls.

- **Systolic Blood Pressure**: pressure against the artery walls when the ventricles contract.
- **Diastolic Blood Pressure**: pressure against the artery walls when the ventricles relax.

When a patient has high blood pressure, it means that they have hypertension. **Hypertension** can lead to serious health concerns including, but not limited to, heart disease, strokes, and irregular heartbeats. Being able to check a patient's blood pressure will enable you to identify if they are at risk, and, from there, proper

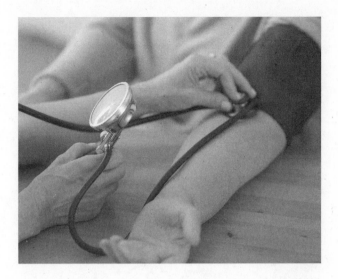

treatments can be performed to try to lower the pressure. A **sphygmomanometer** is used to measure the blood pressure in an individual, and it measures in millimeters of mercury (mm Hg).

The average blood pressure in a healthy person is 120/80 mm Hg, where 120 is the top number and represents systolic, and 80 is the lower number representing diastolic. Normal pressures can also be below this amount and are only considered too low if health complications start to arise. Extremely low blood pressure is

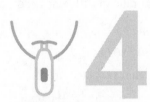

ORAL TEMPERATURE:
Measuring temperature by inserting a thermometer into the mouth. This form of measuring temperature is not as accurate as rectal, temporal, or tympanic, but is more accurate than the axillary method.

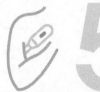

AXILLARY TEMPERATURE:
Measuring temperature by inserting a thermometer into the armpit. This is the least effective in accuracy for measuring temperature. However, the benefit of it is ease of access, especially for taking a quick temperature of a fussy infant.

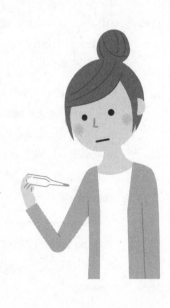

How to use a blood pressure cuff

It is required for all CNAs to be able to use a manual blood pressure cuff. The following are 5 simple steps for measuring blood pressure using a manual cuff:

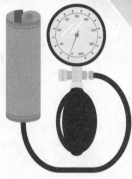

1. Place the proper sized cuff around the patient's upper arm.

2. Place your stethoscope over the brachial artery.

3. Use the black bulb to inflate the cuff until it reaches 180 mm Hg and then turn the silver knob to trap the air.

4. Turn the silver knob again to slowly release the air while watching the dial until you hear a knocking sound. Note that number as it is the systolic pressure.

5. Continue listening until you hear the second knocking sound. This is the diastolic pressure.

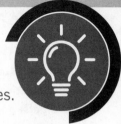

The radial pulse is the most common point to check pulses.

noted as being below 90 for systolic or 60 for diastolic. **Hypertension** is blood pressure 140/90 mm Hg and higher. **Prehypertension** is blood pressure with systolic pressure between 120-139 mm Hg and diastolic pressure between 80-89 mm Hg. As with all vital signs, note accurate numbers in the chart and notify your nurse if a patient goes outside their parameters or has a sudden feeling of dizziness, sweating, or chest pain.

Pulse

The **pulse** of a patient is the rate at which their heart beats, and it is measured in **beats per minute (bpm)**. There are a few different points on the body that can be used to detect and measure a pulse. They are as follows:

- **Carotid Pulse**: in the neck.
- **Brachial Pulse**: at the elbow.
- **Radial Pulse**: on the wrist.
- **Pedal Pulse**: on top of the foot.

To record a patient's pulse, find their radial pulse and count the number of beats that are within 30 seconds, and then multiply that number by two to find the bpm. The average resting heart rate for different age groups:

- **Adults:** 60-100 bpm
- **Kids (1-2 years):** 80-130 bpm
- **Infants (1-11 months):** 80-160 bpm
- **Newborns (under 1 month):** 70-190 bpm

Never use your thumb to check a patient's pulse. You have a pulse in your thumb and will read your own pulse and not the patient's pulse.

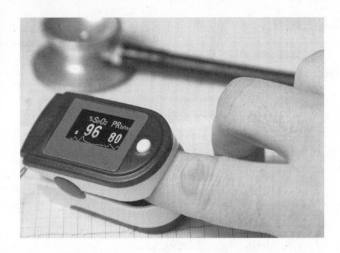

Respiratory Rate

Respiratory rate is the number of breaths a patient takes within a minute. The normal number of breaths per minute for a resting adult is 12-20 breaths, and a breath rate under 12 or over 25 is considered abnormal. Breath rate can vary from patient to patient and depends on their level of recent activity or medication regime. Respiratory rate can be affected due to fever, illnesses, and many other medical complications, so being able to detect and report abnormal breathing is important. Respiration calculation does not require any tools as you will simply watch the rise and fall of the patient's chest. It is important that you pay attention for a full 60 seconds. Each rise counts as a respiration.

Oxygen Saturation

The last vital sign related to the heart and lungs is **oxygen saturation**. This is the level of oxygen found within your body, and dropping levels can indicate serious medical problems. Reading oxygen saturation is almost always part of the routine vital signs taken from a patient. Oxygen is usually measured using an **oximeter**, which can be portable or be a stationary machine.

Each patient will have their own acceptable oxygen range, but a healthy range is between 95%-100%. Anything below 93% should be immediately reported to the nurse as it could indicate something requiring further attention.

Vital Signs Monitor

Some patients in nursing homes and most patients in hospitals and acute care facilities have some type of ongoing monitoring of vitals. These machines record any activity related to a patient's heart and lung functions. These numbers are not only visible in the room but are also visible on a separate screen at the nurses' station. The monitor will alarm if a patient goes outside their personalized parameters, and a CNA may be asked to check on a patient if the vital signs on the monitor change.

The following is an example of the monitor and what the numbers on it mean:

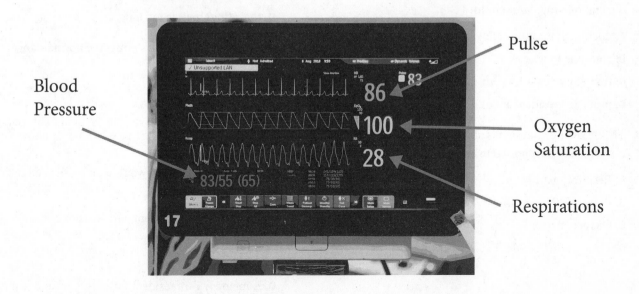

MINI-QUIZ: DATA COLLECTION AND VITAL SIGNS

Directions: Read each question below and choose the correct answer from the four choices provided. Only one choice is correct, so choose carefully.

1. The average, healthy blood pressure is

   A. 90/60 mm Hg.

   B. 140/90 mm Hg.

   C. 120/80 mm Hg.

   D. 105/75 mm Hg.

2. An oral temperature of 99.7°F in an adult should be

   A. rechecked to verify accuracy.

   B. immediately reported to the nurse.

   C. documented in the chart as time allows.

   D. concerning for brain damage.

3. When checking a pulse manually, the preferred location is the

   A. wrist.

   B. neck.

   C. inside of the thigh.

   D. top of the foot.

4. A patient fell earlier, and you observe a bruise during toileting. You should

   A. document it as time allows.

   B. continue to observe it.

   C. immediately notify your nurse.

   D. probe the resident about it.

5. The following vital sign is abnormal and should immediately be reported to the nurse:

   A. Respiration of 16

   B. Pulse of 80 in an adult

   C. Oxygen at 91%

   D. Temperature of 98.9°F

6. A CNA is responsible for tracking and recording which of the following data?

   A. Intake and output

   B. Medication compliance

   C. Medication side effects

   D. Lab results

7. Which of the following complaints should be given to the nurse rather than to the CNA or HHA?

   A. The food is too salty.

   B. The resident is missing a personal item.

   C. The resident's roommate is disrespectful.

   D. The resident stated another CNA abused them.

8. If you check a patient's oxygen saturation with a pulse oximeter and it isn't reading well, you should check to see if

   A. their finger is clean.

   B. they are wearing nail polish.

   C. their finger is too hot.

   D. their fingernail is too long.

9. When you take an adult's pulse, the normal range is

   A. 60-100 bpm.

   B. 80-130 bpm.

   C. 80-160 bpm.

   D. 70-190 bpm.

10. Which of the following would you NOT need to report to the nurse?

    A. A new rash on a patient with sensitive skin

    B. A temperature of 99.4°F

    C. Respiration rate of 10

    D. A memory care resident forgetting what day it is

ANSWER KEY AND EXPLANATIONS

1. C	3. A	5. C	7. D	9. A
2. B	4. C	6. A	8. B	10. D

1. **The correct answer is C.** Average, healthy blood pressure is 120/80 mm Hg. Choice D, 105/75 mm Hg, is considered healthy, but is not the average pressure; 90/60 mm Hg (choice A) is considered low, and 140/90 mm Hg (choice B) is considered too high.

2. **The correct answer is B.** A temperature above 99.0°F is considered a low-grade fever and should be immediately reported to the nurse. You can recheck in the case the patient was doing something that could affect their body temperature (choice A), but it is not automatically required. It should be documented (choice C) but requires immediate notification first. A temperature above 107°F can cause brain damage (choice D).

3. **The correct answer is A.** The preferred manual pulse location is the wrist. If a patient has poor circulation and a weak pulse, the CNA may need to move to the neck (choice B). The thigh (choice C) and the top of the foot (choice D) are usually checked by the nurse or doctor to verify proper circulation.

4. **The correct answer is C.** Any new bruises related to falling should always be reported immediately upon discovery, as they could be related to an injury that has not yet been discovered. You do need to document, but quickly, not as time allows (choice A). You should not simply continue to observe it (choice B) unless it was already reported, and you are instructed to do so by the nurse. Since you know that the patient fell earlier, there is no reason to probe the resident about it at this time (choice D).

5. **The correct answer is C.** An oxygen rate below 93% needs to be reported immediately. The rest of the vital signs are within the normal range.

6. **The correct answer is A.** A CNA must document intake and output, which are related to hydration and kidney, bladder, and bowel function. Medication compliance (choice B) and side effects (choice C) along with lab results (choice D) are all documented by the nurse.

7. **The correct answer is D.** Any suspected or reported abuse must be reported to the nurse, unless the report is about the nurse, in which case the report would go their supervisor. All other choices (A, B, and C) can be reported to the Long-Term Care Ombudsman at the discretion of the resident.

8. **The correct answer is B.** Fingernail polish can interfere with the accuracy of a pulse oximeter. The cleanliness of their finger (choice A), a warm finger (choice C), and the fingernail length (choice D) should not interfere with the reading.

9. **The correct answer is A.** The normal range for a pulse in an adult is 60-100 bpm. 80-130 (choice B) is normal for children over one year of age. 80-160 bpm (choice C) is the normal range for babies one month to 11 months. 70-190 bpm (choice D) is the range for newborns under one month.

10. **The correct answer is D.** A memory care resident is likely to forget what day it is, and thus, this is not needed information. A new rash (choice A) or abnormal vital signs (choices B and C) are all necessary events to report to the nurse.

SUMMING IT UP

- Pathogens are microorganisms that can cause infection. The four main types of pathogens to know are bacteria, virus, fungi, and protozoa.

- The Chain of Infection includes six links and shows how infections begin and spread. Every link must be present for the infection to occur. Infection control breaks at least one link in this chain.

  o The most common way to break the chain is to practice proper and regular handwashing.

  o Handwashing is important for infection control and is the first part of your skills test for the CNA and HHA exam. Wash your hands for at least 20 seconds.

  o If you wash your hands for 19 seconds or less, you will immediately fail the entire exam.

- Safety precautions are in place to ensure that patients and medical personnel resist possible infection. The most important safety precautions to know are universal precautions, standard precautions, and transmission-based precautions.

  o There are seven components to standard precautions: hand hygiene, personal protective equipment (PPE), respiratory hygiene and cough etiquette, environmental cleaning and linens, patient equipment, sharps safety, and waste disposal.

- CNAs and HHAs adhere to proper sterilization and disinfection to prevent the spread of illness or disease. Aides properly handle contaminated items to reduce contact between the items and themselves or anything in their surroundings.

- Every workplace has an emergency preparedness training that you will complete. Emergency preparedness may include shelter in place and/or the RACE method.

- First aid is the immediate and temporary care given to an individual until skilled medical care can be given.

  o If you suspect that a patient is choking, before taking any action, you must ask them if they are choking. If the patient isn't making any sounds or coughing, attempt to expel the lodged object using the Heimlich maneuver.

- Patients may be at risk of falling because of age and fragility, vision quality, poor balance and coordination, unsafe flooring transitions, and clutter.

  o CNAs and HHAs can use bed and chair alarms, lower bed heights, floor mats, aids, shoes and nonslip socks, range of motion exercises, and daily observations to prevent falls.

- Bedrails are present on all hospital beds. The use of bedrails is a form of restraint, which can sometimes further endanger a patient. A patient may also become wedged in a bedrail or wedged between the bedrail and the mattress, which is called entrapment. A head-based bedrail can be engaged to help with transferring out of the bed, repositioning within the bed, and stabilizing after standing up.

- Proper wheelchair use ensures that a patient does not become injured from a fall or collision.

- If patients are wandering in restricted or dangerous areas, they may need redirection, a tracking bracelet, or bed and wheelchair alarms.

- The Occupational Safety and Health Administration (OSHA) is the federal agency that oversees setting and enforcing standard regulations in the workplace. CNAs or HHAs that feel in danger or uncomfortable about a situation while at work should notify the proper individuals. OSHA also dictates the planning, prevention, and disposal of blood-borne pathogens.

- CNAs and HHAs are responsible for collecting data on patients and checking their vital signs throughout each day using questionnaires, intake and output (I & O), assessments, lab tests, observation, and monitoring.

- CNAs and HHAs monitor vital signs including temperature, blood pressure, pulse, respiratory rate, and oxygen saturation.

  o The normal temperature range is 97°-99° Fahrenheit for adults.

  o The average blood pressure in a healthy person is 120/80 mm Hg.

  o Normal pulse rate in an adult is 60-100 bpm.

  o The normal number of breaths per minute for a resting adult is 12-20 breaths.

  o A healthy range of oxygen saturation is between 95%-100%. Anything below 93% should be immediately reported to the nurse.

- A vital signs monitor records any activity related to a patient's heart and lung functions. The monitor will alarm if a patient goes outside their personalized parameters.

PSYCHOSOCIAL CARE SKILLS

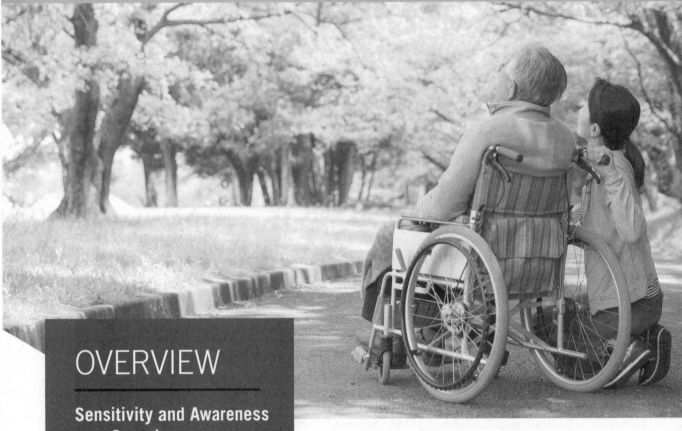

OVERVIEW

SENSITIVITY AND AWARENESS AS A CAREGIVER

As a caregiver, your ability to observe and communicate clearly (and with sensitivity) is important for your success in your CNA or HHA role. Whether you're asking a resident a question or you're simply noticing a change in their behavior, you are employing important verbal and nonverbal skills of communicating and listening. These skills become even more important after you've cared for patients for some time and begin to understand their "normal" behaviors or demeanor. This can help you determine later if a patient seems "off" and alert you to investigate further.

Good communication and observation skills are also key when you're caring for patients whose religious or cultural norms require you to be more sensitive in ways you interact with them or even what medications you distribute to them. In this chapter we'll discuss how caring for patients with mental health and cultural sensitivities can be done effectively with clear communication and education about their unique situations.

MENTAL HEALTH

Mental health encapsulates a person's emotional, psychological, and social conditions, and it can heavily affect their physical health, understanding, compliance, and day-to-day interactions.

This section will cover the following topics to provide a solid foundation regarding mental health for the CNA and HHA:

- Stages of Grief
- Anxiety
- Depression
- Bipolar Disorder and Schizophrenia
- Suicidal Thoughts
- Dementia
- Treatment

Stages of Grief

The **Stages of Grief** are important for a CNA and HHA to understand because many of the patients you encounter are experiencing some type of grief. Patients may be at different stages of grief as they process the loss of their health, mobility, family, home, and even their daily way of life. Grief can be especially present in those living in long-term care facilities as they transition from independent life to medically facilitated, dependent living. It can be deeply traumatic to patients when they are suffering the loss of so many personal freedoms at the same time.

The 5 Stages of Grief

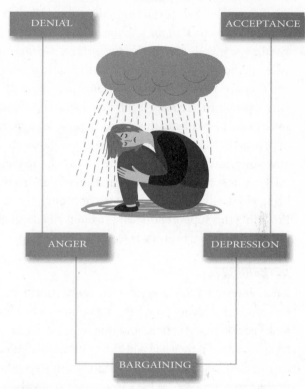

Denial

This stage helps you survive the loss or trauma as you keep the trauma at bay, and your mind tries to deal with the devastating information. You operate under a preferred reality as you try to deny actual reality. This stage protects your mind and body from emotional overload and helps you process the loss and begin adjusting to the loss. In addition to denial, grief can also present as shock at this stage as well.

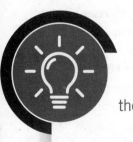

Although this illustration shows a clear descent and ascent within the grief cycle, a patient does NOT necessarily progress in a specific order through each stage. They can, and often do, move back and forth between stages as they continue to process grief.

Anger

Beyond denial is a place of anger. The anger stage can include moments where you blame others, lash out, and have increasingly negative thoughts. Anger allows the person to verbally express opinions about the loss or trauma, whereas, in the previous stage, the goal is to avoid any conversation. In the anger stage, patients are aware of the loss, they are present in their actual reality, and they are extremely frustrated and upset about it. Often, people in this stage feel isolated and alone, and some people never leave this stage. To provide support to patients at this stage, it is important to validate their anger by genuinely listening to them and helping them safely express themselves (helping them refrain from being physically destructive, not cursing loudly, etc.). Providing this support also helps to build and develop a rapport with them over time.

Bargaining

Another term for this is *negotiation*. Some people may bargain with a higher power through prayer. Some may look back on past decisions and wonder what might have happened if they had a healthier diet, took better care of their body, etc. Typically, during this stage, the person grieving asks, "What can I change to get the outcome I want?" The difficult answer is: nothing. The loss or trauma has already occurred, and no amount of bargaining will change that.

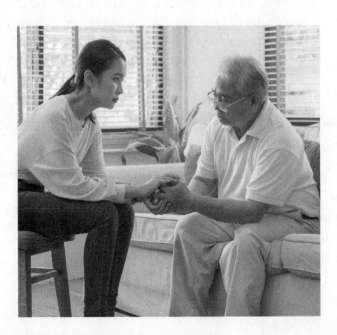

Depression

Depression is the most well-known stage of grief. At this stage the initial feelings of shock and/or anger begin to subside and sadness and the feeling of loss truly take over. This can be one of the most difficult stages, and it can be compounded by the fact many people withdraw inward in reaction to these new and difficult feelings. Because of this, it is important to continue to communicate effectively and patiently with the grieving client. People often assume that a loved one immediately goes into depression without progressing through any other stages along the way. While this can be possible, it is important to understand the other stages can precede or follow this stage.

Acceptance

This is the goal of the stages of grief. While they may not like what has happened and are deeply saddened and even angered by the loss, the patient has accepted it as fact, and emotions begin to stabilize. At this point, good days are more frequent than bad days, but the patient is by no means simply "over" the loss. Instead, the person has found their new normal through acceptance.

Anxiety

Anxiety is something that everyone experiences at some point in their lives. It stems from high-stress situations, and, for the everyday person, this stress can result from events like giving a presentation or working on an unfamiliar project. Normal anxiety is usually infrequent or intermittent and occurs in situations that we expect them to, like ones that bring about stress or worry.

However when anxiety is recurring, irrational, and interferes with their everyday living, a person suffers from what's called an **anxiety disorder**. Anxiety disorders can take on many different forms that affect daily life, and they cannot be controlled easily. Often, a patient's stress response may be out of proportion to the situation if they have an anxiety disorder. In addition, anxiety is often irrational and can occur "out of nowhere," thus making cares more difficult. As you get to know your patients, you may become aware of anxiety triggers (such as allergies, fear of transfers, etc.) that can help you provide better care and decrease anxiety.

People can also be affected by more than one anxiety disorder at one time, and there are many different types of anxiety to be familiar with as a nurse's aide. **Generalized anxiety** stems from any kind of stress that the individual may experience, and its triggers are not always easy to identify. Individuals with **panic anxiety** experience spontaneous panic attacks that cause them to lose touch with reality, become hyperactive, and lose the ability to problem-solve. Patients may complain of medical symptoms such as a racing heart, numbness, tingling, and sweating. Those with **social anxiety** become disproportionally stressed and experience panic attacks when dealing with or anticipating social interactions. This type of anxiety can also be called social phobia. People with social anxiety are often very reluctant to leave their rooms, eat in the cafeteria, or participate in group activities. Individuals with **separation anxiety** experience major distress when anticipating or while being separated from home and loved ones. Separation can also cause paranoia in the individual—they fear they will lose a loved one or that something bad will happen to them when they leave. Separation anxiety can be heightened, often extremely, upon admission to a long-term care facility, especially if a resident had to leave their spouse or other loved one who they lived with.

A **phobia** is an anxiety disorder that causes an individual to have irrational fear of something. Phobias can develop over many elements of their care—fear of needles, blood, allergic reactions, and heights (like when you're using a lift to move them). Often, care situations arise where the patient must face the phobia, and it can cause panic in the person. One common example of this is a person who has a fear of enclosed spaces (claustrophobia), and they need an MRI. The test is conducted within a very tight space, and it can cause increased anxiety.

As a CNA, it's important for you to remember that a person who suffers from any anxiety disorder (or multiple disorders) should avoid coffee, chocolate, and alcohol because these substances can increase anxiety. Another way you can help patients combat anxiety is

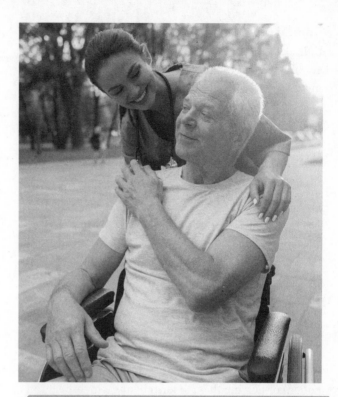

> People can also be affected by more than one anxiety disorder at one time, and there are many different types of anxiety to be familiar with as a nurse's aide.

to help them exercise in whatever way they can, as this releases endorphins which are naturally occurring chemicals in the body that help calm anxiety and stress.

Depression

The term *depression* is often overused to describe anyone that is feeling sorrow or apathy during a period of their life. However, **depression** is defined as a persistent feeling of sadness and lack of regard for many things, and it can affect how someone thinks, feels, and behaves. Much like anxiety, depression can become a major problem and often affects how an individual functions in their day-to-day life.

Clinical depression affects an individual's daily functions. Clinical depression is also called **major depressive disorder**. Symptoms from clinical depression include, but are not limited to:

- Feelings of sadness, emptiness, or unworthiness
- Being easily frustrated or angered
- Having no interest in things that the individual usually enjoys
- Low energy or significant effort is required to complete any task
- Large increase or decrease in appetite
- Suicidal thoughts or tendencies
- Anxiety

It is important for you to report any changes in behavior in a patient. When a patient is depressed, it is important for your to communicate effectively and listen empathetically. Spending more time with the patient or helping them to form bonds with others can help alleviate their worries. Thoughtful interactions and encouragement can go a long way in helping the patient feel better.

Bipolar Disorder and Schizophrenia

Both bipolar disorder and schizophrenia can be extremely debilitating and a lifelong struggle. As a care provider, it is important for you to be aware of these illnesses and what the doctors and nurses may request you to document as a tool for illness management. We will define and discuss these conditions in this section.

First, here are some important terms to know about these conditions. If a patient is **delusional**, they are out of touch with reality and believe in something that is not true. Even if the facts show that something is not

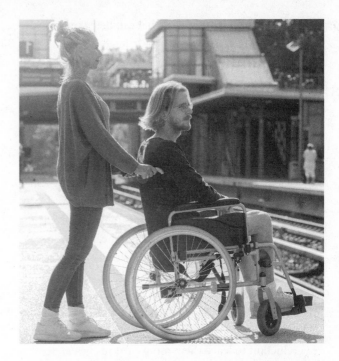

true, a delusional person will alter reality in their mind to make it true to them. Delusion is often a symptom of a disorder (such as schizophrenia) and is sometimes paired with paranoia as well. Do not try to rationalize with a delusional person. This can be unsafe. Best practice is to allow that person their delusion and try to guide them to a safe place while seeking help from the charge nurse. A patient experiencing **paranoia** is highly suspicious of people and situations, and they can fully believe they are being persecuted when they are not. Paranoia is often a symptom of a disorder (such as schizophrenia) and is sometimes paired with delusion.

A **hallucination** is the presence of something that is not present in reality. It can manifest as affecting only one of the five senses or across multiple senses. Most hallucinations are visual (seeing a person or animal) or

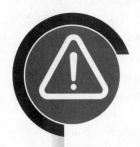

Alert! A urinary tract infection can cause mood shifts and delusions in the older population. Report and document any unusual behavior patterns ASAP to your charge nurse.

auditory (hearing voices that tell you to do something dangerous or harmful). However, hallucinations can also be olfactory (affecting smell, such as smelling feces at all times) or gustatory (affecting taste, such as only tasting rotting food, even if it's fresh). Hallucinations related to mental illness are often scary, violent, and degrading to the patient. Although it is possible to have positive hallucinations, it is important to understand that this is an exception, not a standard.

Bipolar Disorder

Bipolar disorder is a mood disorder that is characterized by "highs," called **mania**, and "lows," called **depression**. Mania is a grandiose feeling of euphoria, confidence, and talkativeness coupled with increased activity, decreased need for sleep, and racing thoughts. Depression is an intense feeling of sorrow, apathy, and grief. This can also manifest as anger, and the patient can lash out. Appetite, sleep, and anxiety all increase. A person with bipolar disorder will experience mood swings resulting in very unstable periods of mania and depression, and some patients may also experience hallucinations. These swings are unpredictable, and, at times, a patient may need a higher level of care than your workplace can provide.

Schizophrenia

Schizophrenia is a biologically based disorder that affects a person's perception and understanding of reality. One of the hardest struggles for those living with schizophrenia is **disorganized thoughts** as the illness does not allow them to think in an organized fashion, even if they are extremely intelligent. Current medications also do not address this symptom. Keep this in mind when providing instructions or asking for feedback from a patient with schizophrenia. The more frustrated they become, the more their symptoms can increase. Some patients with schizophrenia may experience paranoia, delusions, and hallucinations. Pay attention to a patient who says they always smell or taste strong odors or flavors as this can be a type of hallucination. Document this observation if you notice that it is an ongoing issue, regardless of the smell or taste that is present. Keep in mind that patients with schizophrenia may have all or a combination of the symptoms mentioned above.

Suicidal Thoughts

Suicidal thoughts, or thoughts of taking one's own life, are extreme reactions to stress and depression. As a caregiver of someone having suicidal thoughts, you should not take those expressions lightly. People who are having suicidal thoughts often feel that there is

Suicide warning signs include but are not limited to:

Talking about or referencing suicide

Attaining the means to take one's own life

Feeling trapped, hopeless, or meaningless

Heightened use of alcohol or drugs

Committing actions that are dangerous or self-destructive

Reclusiveness or avoiding social interaction

Giving away belongings for no apparent reason

Saying goodbye as if it were for the last time

SYMPTOMS OF DEMENTIA BY TYPE		
VASCULAR DEMENTIA	**LEWY BODY DEMENTIA**	**ALZHEIMER'S DISEASE**
Memory, cognition, and communication are all affected		
Affects ability to problem solve and reason first		Affects ability to store new information via memories first
Hallucination can occur, but not guaranteed	Early onset of hallucinations	Hallucinations occur after several years
Sleep disorder not noted	REM sleep disorder	Sleep issues vary by patient
Limited movements develop alongside cognitive changes	Shaky movements common	Cognitive decline occurs before physical decline

no other solution to their problems or that the future holds nothing for them. A family history of suicide can also impress upon a person and influence their decision. These thoughts most commonly stem from severe depression, but just because an individual is not depressed does not mean they cannot be suicidal. When a patient is admitted to a psychiatric unit, the top priority and main concern in their report is whether they have suicidal thoughts or tendencies.

If you or anyone you know is having suicidal thoughts, please seek immediate help and professional treatment as soon as possible. If you can't find immediate help, you should contact the U.S. National Suicide Prevention Lifeline at (800)-273-8255 or via online chat at **https://suicidepreventionlifeline.org**

Dementia

One important and common area of mental health among older populations is **dementia**, which is a catch-all term for various memory and cognitive-affecting disorders. All forms of dementia have a biological source, and dementia can be short-term (as a result of an infection or traumatic event) and long-term (such as Alzheimer's disease, which is degenerative).

There are three most common types of dementia. **Vascular dementia** is caused by damaged blood vessels and is often associated with unhealthy behavior over a period of time. Some common behaviors contributing to vascular dementia include smoking, heavy drinking, eating a poor diet, having heart disease, and

suffering prior strokes. **Lewy body dementia** is caused by microscopic deposits in the brain that damage brain cells slowly over time. **Alzheimer's disease** is caused by a slow, progressive death of nerves and loss of brain tissue. The brain shrinks dramatically, and, eventually, all functions, even basic ones such as swallowing, are affected.

Treatments

For patients who suffer from mental illness, a **psychiatrist** performs an assessment of the patient and diagnoses their illness. The psychiatrist also prescribes appropriate medicine for the patient. Psychiatrists are medical doctors that specialize in mental health and substance use disorders (such as a substance addiction). They are not the same as a **psychologist**. Without supervision, psychologists do not have the power to write a prescription for patients or clients like a psychiatrist does. However, psychologists do have more targeted training in communication techniques and ongoing therapy, so they are often used when a patient does not want to use a medication to help their mental illness and would rather have someone to talk to and listen to them. Also, therapists and counselors may be added to a patient's care plan for ongoing therapy in addition to the medications prescribed.

As a nurse's aide, you can use several strategies and tactics when caring for patients with mental illness. **Active listening** is an essential communication skill to have when dealing with mental health because hearing what the patient has to say is important. Truly listening, understanding what they have to say, and allowing them to feel heard is called **validation** and is an extremely useful tool in this type of situation. You do not have to agree with what they are saying to validate their feelings. People that suffer from major mental illnesses and dementia often feel misunderstood and alone. It is out of your scope of practice to try and "help" your patient, but you can show them **compassion.** Lending a listening ear, avoiding judgement regarding delusions, and resisting the urge to "defend" paranoid thoughts are all useful tools for building better rapport with patients who have mental illness and dementia. **Distraction** is an extremely useful tool for those living with schizophrenia and varying levels of dementia. The mind will grow whatever topic it is fed. If you simply move the conversation to something neutral, such as the weather or the next meal, a person that is paranoid or confused will often follow you willingly into the new conversation.

Treatments for mental health are great in variety depending on the person and disorder. Some treatments are simple where only medication is prescribed to the patient, and others require a mixture of medication and therapy. **Medications** are used to relieve the symptoms of a mental disorder or condition. They are prescribed by psychiatrists and mostly go together with therapy and programs. Medications are rarely stand-alone treatments for mental health. **Therapy** is used to not only help the psychiatrist or psychologist diagnose the patient but also allow the patient to give their point of view and share things that they hold back from other people. This also can empower the patient to realize the steps they need to take to better themselves and work toward a stronger state of mental health.

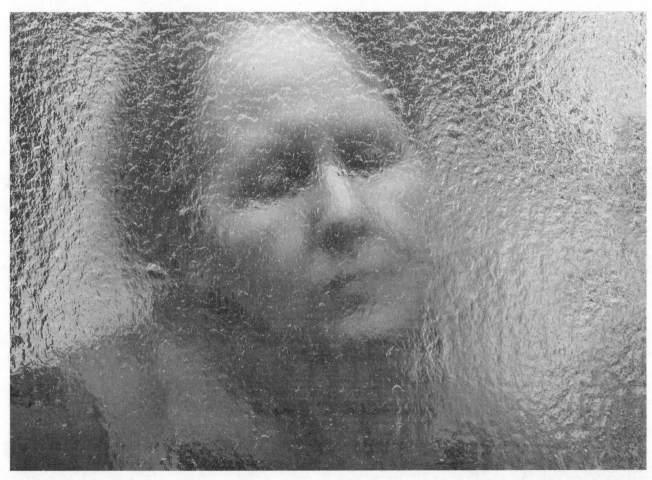

MINI-QUIZ: MENTAL HEALTH

Directions: Read each question below and choose the correct answer from the four choices provided. Only one choice is correct, so choose carefully.

1. A psychiatrist provides

   A. therapy to mentally ill patients.

   B. medication to mentally ill patients.

   C. legal oversight to those working with mentally ill patients.

   D. Choices A and B

2. A type of anxiety that is related to irrational fear of enclosed places is a type of

   A. generalized anxiety.

   B. panic disorder.

   C. phobia.

   D. social anxiety.

3. A patient reports a strong and persistent smell of feces without a source. They may be experiencing which of the following?

   A. Delusions

   B. Hallucinations

   C. Paranoia

   D. Mania

4. If a patient's mood shifts dramatically from the beginning of the shift to the end of the shift, they may suffer from

   A. anxiety.

   B. depression.

   C. bipolar disorder.

   D. schizophrenia.

5. A male patient seems very uninterested in daily cares and refuses to attend any activities, stating they are all boring and he doesn't care about much anymore. He may be experiencing which mental health concern?

   A. Social anxiety

   B. Depression

   C. Dementia

   D. Schizophrenia

6. The stage of grief connected to blame and lashing out is

   A. denial.

   B. anger.

   C. bargaining.

   D. depression.

7. The stage of grief that protects your body and mind from overload immediately following a loss or trauma is

   A. denial.

   B. bargaining.

   C. anger.

   D. acceptance.

8. All of the following are a common sign of suicidal thoughts EXCEPT:

   A. Saying goodbye as if it is final

   B. Hallucinations

   C. Getting rid of personal belongings

   D. Talking about a plan for harming oneself

9. A useful tool for helping a person that is having a delusional experience is to

   A. help them get in touch with reality.

   B. point out what is wrong with their thinking.

   C. distract them by bringing up another neutral subject.

   D. encourage them to share more about their delusion.

10. Which type of dementia is related to the slow shrinking of the brain?

    A. Lewy body dementia

    B. Vascular dementia

    C. Alzheimer's disease

    D. None of these

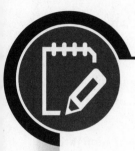

NOTES

ANSWER KEY AND EXPLANATIONS

1. D	3. B	5. B	7. A	9. C
2. C	4. C	6. B	8. B	10. C

1. **The correct answer is D.** Although a psychiatrist is usually the main prescriber of medications for mentally ill patients, they can, and sometimes do, provide therapy as well. They are not responsible for the legal oversight of patient care (choice C).

2. **The correct answer is C.** Phobias are a type of anxiety that directly result from a specific fear of something or someone. Generalized anxiety (choice A) does not have a specific root cause. Panic disorder (choice B) is not solely triggered by a fear of something or someone. Social anxiety (choice D) is related to crowded or public places.

3. **The correct answer is B.** Hallucinations can occur across all 5 senses. Delusion (choice A) is the perception of something happening that is not in reality. Paranoia (choice C) is an unrealistic fear that you are being watched, followed, or targeted in some negative way. Mania (choice D) is a heightened state of euphoria associated with bipolar disorder.

4. **The correct answer is C.** Dramatic shifts of mood are often a hallmark sign of bipolar disorder. Although they can be present with anxiety (choice A) and schizophrenia (choice D), they are not as common. Dramatic mood swings are not usually associated with depression (choice B).

5. **The correct answer is B.** This patient is showing apathy, which is a common symptom associated with depression. He does not express any apprehension about going to activities, so it is unlikely that he is experiencing social anxiety (choice A). He does not show any signs of delusions, paranoia, or disorganized thought, so schizophrenia is unlikely (choice D). His memory and problem-solving skills are not in question here, so dementia is also unlikely (choice C).

6. **The correct answer is B.** Although blame and lashing out can also occur in depression (choice D) it is most seen in the anger stage. Denial (choice A) and bargaining (choice C) are not associated with these actions.

7. **The correct answer is A.** Denial is typically the first stage of grief and is the result of information overload immediately after a diagnosis, loss, etc. Bargaining, anger, and acceptance (choices B, C, and D) are not related to protecting your body and mind from overload.

8. **The correct answer is B.** Hallucinations are not commonly considered to be a sign of suicidal thoughts. All other choices are directly connected to this.

9. **The correct answer is C.** An extremely useful tool for interacting with a delusional person is the method of distraction. This can allow them to focus on a neutral subject that does not upset them. Helping them get in touch with reality (choice A) or pointing out what is wrong with their thinking (choice B) can only agitate the situation. Encouraging them to share more about their delusion (choice D) will only validate their thinking.

10. **The correct answer is C.** Alzheimer's disease is the only type of dementia that is related to the slow shrinking of the brain. Lewy body dementia (choice A) is the result of microscopic deposits in the brain. Vascular dementia (choice B) is the result of physical health decline, such as heart disease.

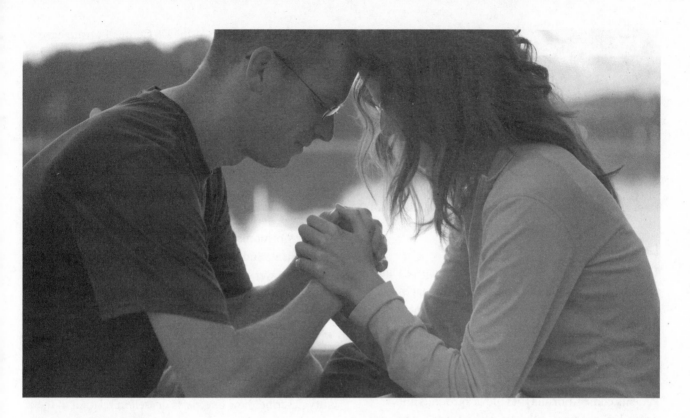

CULTURAL AND SPIRITUAL NEEDS

This section will cover cultural competence, including a patient's basic cultural and spiritual needs, and will provide some examples of how to improve cultural competence in a medical facility.

Cultural Competence

As a nurse's aide, it is important to understand a patient's cultural and spiritual needs to provide compassionate and effective care. **Cultural competence** is the ability to provide care that matches the cultural, social, and spiritual requirements and expectations of the patient and their family. Healthcare professionals take care of the whole person, including the body, mind, and spirit. Practicing cultural competence will enable you to treat patients better and allow them and their families to feel comfortable and validated, making your job easier in caring for them.

The cultural needs of a patient may include, but are not limited to, factors such as ethnicity, gender, language, mental ability, nationality, race, religion, sexuality, and socioeconomic status. We will define each of these

factors and then discuss best practices for caring for patients with these needs.

Ethnicity

Ethnicity relates to either a particular region or a specific cultural tradition. Examples of ethnicity include Hispanic, Arabic, and Han Chinese populations. While people of the same ethnicities may share a common language, religion, or cultural tradition, they are often present in a variety of locations.

Gender

Gender is more nuanced than simply male and female, and it is important to be familiar with various other gender identities. Someone who is **transgender**, for example, identifies as a gender different from their assumed gender at birth. Someone with a **non-binary** gender identity does not define their gender based on the gender binary of male-female. Instead, they may identify as between genders, beyond gender, or gender neutral. Someone who is **gender neutral** does not identify as male or female but as neutral with no need for a gender label.

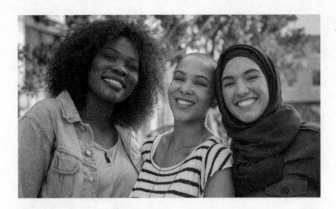

Language

This includes both oral and written language. In addition, there are varying dialects within languages, such as Mexican Spanish and Spanish derived from Spain. It is important to gather clarity on what their language preference is, both spoken and in writing.

Physical and Mental Ability

Patients come from all types of backgrounds and, depending on genetic disorders, their medical history, and current trauma, their physical and mental abilities will vary. This can include mobility and sensory limits, memory loss, mood swings, and difficulty processing information like instructions.

Nationality

This cultural identification is very strong for certain groups, including but not limited to Eastern European countries such as Ukraine, Greece, Romania, etc., Middle Eastern countries such as Saudi Arabia and Pakistan, Asian countries such as India and Japan, and African countries including Senegal, Kenya, and Ghana. Each nationality brings a whole set of cultural contexts that are unique and should be honored whenever possible.

Race

Historically, labels of race have been used to represent major groupings of humans based upon physical characteristics common to certain ancestries. The color of an individual's skin, hair, and eyes have all been seen as racial traits. In recent years, however, self-identification has come to play a larger role in conceptions of race,

and institutions, such as the US Census Bureau, have recognized the role that shared ancestry, national origin, and sociocultural groups have on descriptions of race. The US Census Bureau uses the following labels: American Indian or Alaskan Native, Asian, Black or African American, Native Hawaiian and Other Pacific Islander, and White.

Religion

In the US, the most practiced religions include the following: Christianity (including Protestantism, Catholicism, Mormonism, and Orthodoxy), Islam, Judaism, Hinduism, Buddhism, and Agnosticism (believing in a higher power only).

Sexuality

Sexuality encompasses a broad range of human behaviors including one's sexual orientation and identity. Sexual orientation describes to whom one is attracted, romantically, emotionally, and/or sexually while identity describes how one views oneself in relation to their orientation. Orientations include heterosexual, gay/lesbian, bisexual, asexual, and pansexual (attraction to individuals without consideration of sex or gender), among others.

Socioeconomic Status

The financial background and status of your patient can be an important cultural component of how they identify. One common scenario is a person who came from wealth but cannot sustain that wealth in a long-term care facility. Understanding this can help you appreciate their approach to cares and their loss from a psychological perspective. Not only has their health declined, but they have lost their financial freedom as well.

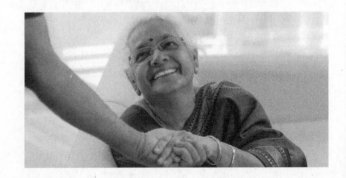

Cultural Needs: Best Practices

Although it is impossible to cover all possible cultural needs that you may encounter, we will review common areas and best practices associated with them to help you as a CNA or HHA. However, it is always your professional responsibility to both read the files and learn from the patients about their cultural needs.

Eye Contact

Although Americans value eye contact as a sign of respect, this is the exact opposite in many cultures. Upon meeting a new patient, it is important to establish their preference before making assumptions. If you feel comfortable, you can ask. You should also make a mental note about the patient's reaction when you make eye contact. For example, the patient might look away or bow their head. These observations can provide valuable information about a patient's needs. A patient's culture and religion can also give insight into their eye contact preferences. For example, in Middle Eastern and Asian cultures and the Muslim faith, direct eye contact is a sign of disrespect.

Gender Preference of Direct Care Providers

Some cultures and religions have strong preferences in which gender performs care. Most that have a religious or cultural need in this area will request or require the same gender as themselves to provide all direct care. Thus, a female patient will request another female and vice versa.

Making Decisions

When a patient has a native language other than English, it is important to use that language during cares and to provide a translator at every meeting. It is also extremely important to honor the cultural and religious backgrounds of families as it pertains to decision-making. Some cultures, including some Native American tribes, have a matriarchal hierarchy, in which women are usually the main decision-makers rather than men. In addition, you should honor the patient's request about who they want to help them make decisions. Patients may also want to include a family member who is not present. You can speak up for the patient if they bring this up to you during cares.

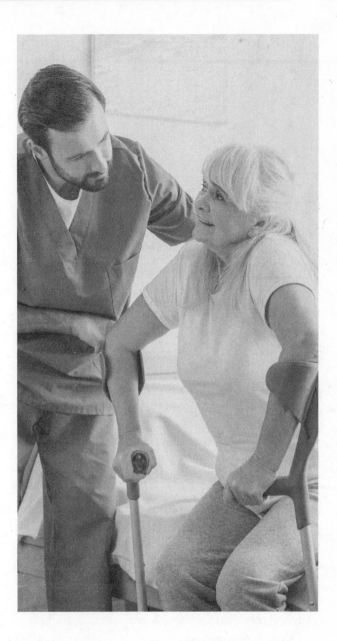

Communication

It is common to have patients that are not able to fully participate in all aspects of their care and decision-making. Your job is to present all directions in an easily understood manner. Clear, simple instructions coupled with hand gestures, demonstrations, and facial expressions are tools that can increase understanding and compliance. It can be scary to be transferred, and it can be humiliating to be cleaned up after an accident. Add confusion to this and the patient can become less and less compliant. Use kindness and compassion as your guide and they will feel much safer.

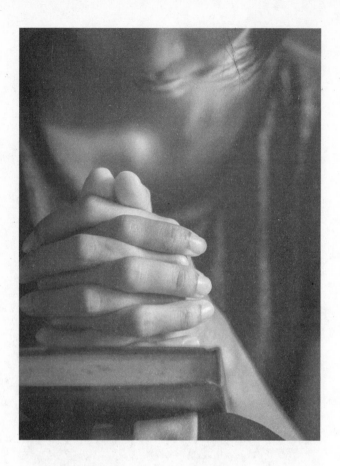

Spiritual Needs: Best Practices

Just as there are numerous cultures, there are also many spiritual and religious backgrounds that you may encounter as a CNA or HHA. It is important to read the chart of every patient you care for, but it is equally important to communicate directly with them to get to know them and their spiritual needs. The following are common topics across multiple religions and can help you when providing care.

Clothing

This area allows for a variety of spiritual needs. Some religions, such as Islam, may always require head coverings for women when they encounter someone outside of their home. Judaism requires head coverings for both men and women. Some religions, like Mormonism, require special undergarments to be worn at all times. Some faiths may dictate the type of clothing, such as dresses or skirts only, long sleeve shirts, or no decolletage showing, as is often seen in Amish or Mennonite faith backgrounds.

Diet

Restrictions are common within a variety of religions. Judaism does not allow for the mixing of dairy and meat; thus, a patient will need food prepared in kosher kitchens or without the combination of the two on their plate. Judaism and Islam do not permit any type of consumption of pork either. The majority of Hindus are vegetarian, avoiding both meat and eggs; for those who do consume meat, red meat is often limited to lamb and goat as cows are viewed as sacred. During the season of Lent, Catholics do not eat meat on Fridays. Similarly, Orthodox Christians avoid meat, fish, and dairy products on Wednesdays and Fridays, in addition to other fasting periods throughout the year. This must be noted on their charts so medical personnel and the dietary department can make arrangements.

Medical Practices

Some religions have clear guidelines on the type of medical treatments that are allowed or restricted. For example, Jehovah's Witnesses choose not to receive blood, even in cases of imminent death. In addition, some religions prefer alternative medicine, such as homeopathic doctors, spiritual healers, and acupuncture. This is seen at times in Native American spirituality, New Ageism, and Eastern cultures.

Spiritual Practice

Different religions have different needs for their worship. Christians often attend a service on Sundays and communion may or may not be brought in by an outside priest or church member. Muslims pray five times a day and must face toward Mecca (easterly in the US). Those that are agnostic and spiritual, rather than connected to a specific religion, may wish to meditate, burn incense, or chant. Spiritual practices are both connected to religions and deeply personal. Never assume that you know a patient's preferences because you know their spiritual background. Always discuss this with the patient and allow for spiritual time throughout each day as needed and requested. It may mean that you need to adjust your schedule, but it is important to honor their needs.

Providing Culturally Competent Care

Many medical facilities are working toward stronger competence throughout all aspects of patient interaction, and there are many ways they are doing so. There are several ways to maximize cultural competence in a medical facility, and the following are some examples. Please note that this is not the limit of methods that can be used, and it is important for you to know your patients and work toward increasing your rapport with them. This will also help to increase your cultural competence.

Encourage Family Involvement

It can take a toll on the patient when their family members aren't included in day-to-day care. Having the support of their loved ones can help patients make the best decisions for themselves and bring them comfort. It is equally important to respect the patient's preference on which family members can be involved. The voice of the patient should always be heard and respected.

Training in Cultural Competence

Medical facilities training their staff to have a stronger cultural competence will better enable them to recognize and work with patient's values and beliefs. This will also help the staff be more aware of the nuances of their own culture and allow the caregiver to be aware of how it can influence or conflict with a patient's culture.

Diversified Staff

Employing people from diversified cultures throughout a facility will help to provide support to a patient in a similar way to encouraging family involvement. There is comfort found in dealing with people of the same or similar culture as you. Being able to provide a diversified staff that aligns with the patients' cultural and spiritual needs is extremely beneficial.

Interpreter Services

Being able to access an interpreter will make communication much more efficient for both the staff and the patient.

Traditional Healers

Some facilities allow a patient to reference or utilize a traditional healer if it suits them. At times, a patient may refuse any kind of treatment that is not done so in a traditional manner.

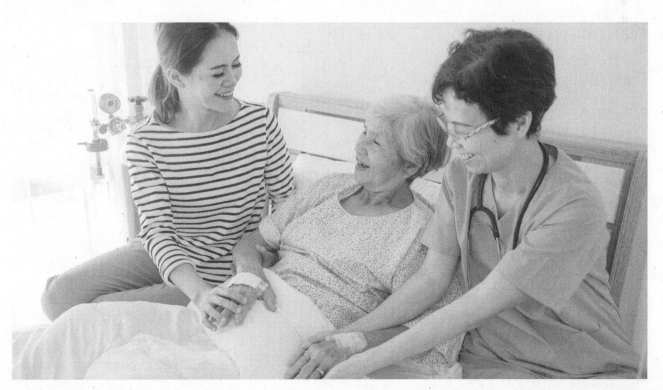

MINI-QUIZ: CULTURAL AND SPIRITUAL NEEDS

Directions: Read each question below and choose the correct answer from the four choices provided. Only one choice is correct, so choose carefully.

1. The term that describes a person who does not identify as one specific gender is

   A. transgender.

   B. non-binary.

   C. gender neutral.

   D. male.

2. Judaism does not permit the mixing of

   A. milk and meat.

   B. dairy and meat.

   C. dairy and pork.

   D. milk and pork.

3. If a Muslim patient wants to attend to their spiritual and cultural needs, they will likely need time in their schedule to

   A. light candles and incense.

   B. pray five times a day.

   C. take communion.

   D. watch religious services online or on TV.

4. A person that romantically prefers the same gender as themselves is

   A. heterosexual.

   B. gay or lesbian.

   C. bisexual.

   D. pansexual.

5. One way to help a patient with cognitive deficits is to

   A. speak loudly so they can hear you better.

   B. write everything down so they can read what you are doing.

   C. meet with the family to have them interpret what you are saying.

   D. use simple instructions coupled with hand gestures to explain cares.

6. A Native American resident must make an important decision. They've told you that the tribe they were raised in has a matriarchal structure. Based on this information, who will most likely be the best person to help them make this decision?

   A. Their lawyer

   B. Their female relative

   C. Their male relative

   D. There is no cultural preference.

7. A resident just moved in and wants to hang a prominent flag of his home country of Pakistan above his bed. This is an example of

   A. patriotism.

   B. religion.

   C. spiritualism.

   D. ethnicity.

8. You note on a patient's care plan that Chinese is their native language. When seeking an interpreter to help you, it is helpful to

A. choose the first person you can find so the resident is not waiting long.

B. note what region they come from as different regions have different dialects.

C. ask a Chinese-speaking coworker to take over their care.

D. ask the charge nurse for help.

9. A staff member provides excellent care but is the opposite gender of a new resident whose culture has restrictions on interactions between different genders. Cultural best practices would encourage the staff member to

A. continue to provide care due to their experience and high quality of work.

B. request a coworker of the same gender as the resident be assigned for care.

C. confront the resident about their gender preferences.

D. work with the resident until they refuse care.

10. An Asian male resident is being transferred from another facility, and you are asked to document his mood. You notice his head is frequently down when you are talking to him, although he communicates in an upbeat, respectful manner. How should you document this?

A. He is depressed because he will not make eye contact.

B. He could be depressed because he never looks up.

C. He is upbeat and positive, and his lack of eye contact is culturally appropriate.

D. He is upbeat and positive, but his lack of eye contact is culturally inappropriate.

ANSWER KEY AND EXPLANATIONS

1. C	3. B	5. D	7. A	9. B
2. B	4. B	6. B	8. B	10. C

1. **The correct answer is C.** Gender neutral refers to a person that does not identify with one specific gender. Transgender (choice A) refers to a person that identifies as the opposite gender than the one assigned to them at birth. Non-binary (choice B) refers to a person that identifies with a gender or combination of genders outside of solely male or female. Male (choice D) is a traditional gender assignment.

2. **The correct answer is B.** Judaism does not permit the mixing of any dairy and meat, not just milk (choice A). Judaism does not permit the consumption of pork at all (choices C and D).

3. **The correct answer is B.** Muslims pray five times a day, and time must be provided for a patient to do so. Lighting candles and incense (choice A) is not required. Muslims do not take communion (choice C). While they may watch religious services online or on TV (choice D), it is not a required part of their daily prayer needs.

4. **The correct answer is B.** Gay or lesbian refers to people that romantically prefer those of the same gender. Heterosexual (choice A) refers to people that romantically prefer members of the opposite gender. Bisexual (choice C) people prefer both genders, and pansexual (choice D) people do not have a gender preference.

5. **The correct answer is D.** People with cognitive deficits respond well to simple instructions coupled with hand gestures. This helps to reduce any misunderstandings. Speaking loudly (choice A) and writing everything down (choice B) will not increase comprehension. In addition, meeting with the family (choice C) can be helpful but not always.

6. **The correct answer is B.** Some Native American cultures are matriarchal in structure, meaning women play a key role in decision-making. As such, the resident might consult a female relative. While a lawyer (choice A) and a male relative (choice C) may also be present, they are not the most important for the resident. Choice D is incorrect and culturally insensitive.

7. **The correct answer is A.** Patriotism ties directly back to the country of origin. The country of Pakistan is not a religion (choice B) or a spiritualism (choice C). Pakistan has an ethnically diverse population, and as only the country is referenced, ethnicity (choice D) is not a factor.

8. **The correct answer is B.** China is home to a variety of languages, each with their own dialects. An interpreter with a different dialect than the speaker can impede communication and create issues in any setting, let alone medical care. Choosing the first person you can find (choice A) and asking the charge nurse for help (choice D) do not address the ongoing language barrier. In addition, asking a Chinese coworker to take over their care (choice C) is insensitive and does not ensure that the correct language is known.

9. **The correct answer is B.** Using known cultural needs to make decisions for a resident's care is a culturally competent choice. Instigating a confrontation (choice C) or expecting the resident to speak up after care has already started (choice D) does not serve their needs. To simply provide care knowing their cultural background (choice A) is culturally insensitive.

10. **The correct answer is C.** In many Asian cultures, bowing the head is a sign of respect. His mannerisms are in line with a happy and mentally healthy individual in every other way. Choices A, B, and D are incorrect.

SUMMING IT UP

- Mental health is a person's emotional, psychological, and social conditions, and it can affect their physical health, understanding, compliance, and day-to-day interactions.

- Patients grieve when they experience a loss. The stages of grief include denial, anger, bargaining, depression, and acceptance.

- Anxiety stems from high-stress situations.

  - Anxiety disorders result from feelings of anxiety that become frequent and powerful, including generalized anxiety, panic anxiety, social anxiety, separation anxiety, and phobias.

- Depression is a persistent feeling of sadness and lack of regard for many things, and it can affect how an individual functions in their day-to-day life.

- Bipolar disorder is a mood disorder that is characterized by "highs," called mania, and "lows," called depression.

  - Mania is a grandiose feeling of euphoria, confidence, and talkativeness coupled with increased activity, decreased need for sleep, and racing thoughts. Depression is an intense feeling of sorrow, apathy, and grief.

- Schizophrenia is a biologically based disorder that affects a person's perception and understanding of reality. It can include disorganized thoughts, paranoia, delusions, and hallucinations.

- Suicidal thoughts, or thoughts of taking one's own life, are extreme reactions to stress and depression.

- Dementia includes various memory and cognitive-affecting disorders like vascular dementia, Lewy body dementia, and Alzheimer's disease.

- A patient with mental illness may be treated by a psychiatrist or psychologist, and treatment may include medication or therapy. As a CNA or HHA, it is important to be an active listener and show compassion to patients with mental illness.

- Cultural competence is the ability to provide care that matches the cultural, social, and spiritual requirements and expectations of the patient and their family.

  - A patient's cultural and social needs may stem from their ethnicity, gender, language, mental ability, nationality, race, religion, sexuality, and socioeconomic status.

- Areas to consider when providing culturally competent care include eye contact, gender preference of care providers, communication, and cognitive deficits.

- A patient's spiritual needs may affect their clothing, diet, medical procedures, and spiritual practices.

- There are many ways to provide culturally competent care including encouraging family involvement, training in cultural competence, having a diversified staff, using interpreter services, and bringing in traditional healers.

PART IV
THREE PRACTICE TESTS

Practice Test 1

Practice Test 2

Practice Test 3

PRACTICE TEST

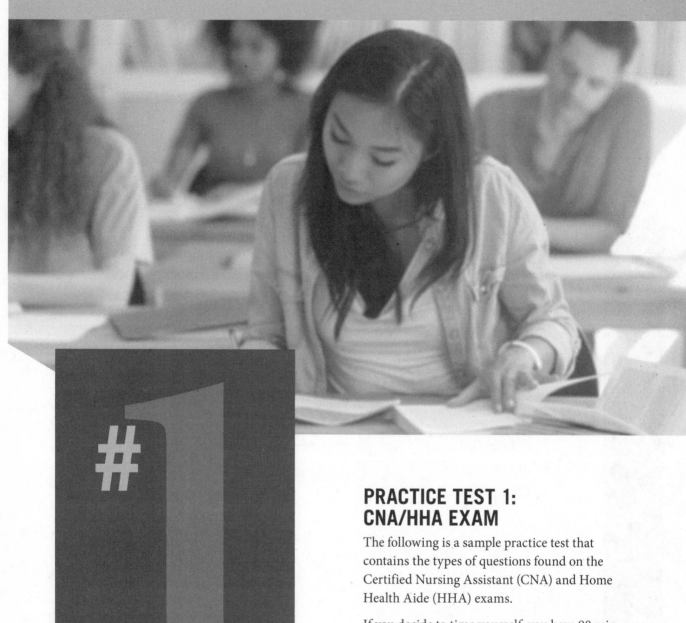

 # 1

PRACTICE TEST 1: CNA/HHA EXAM

The following is a sample practice test that contains the types of questions found on the Certified Nursing Assistant (CNA) and Home Health Aide (HHA) exams.

If you decide to time yourself, you have 90 minutes to complete this practice test. Use this time limit to gauge your comfort level under time constraints and your level of mastery of the types of questions found in the exam.

After you have completed this practice test, check your answers against the answer key and explanations that follow the test.

PRACTICE TEST 1: CNA/HHA EXAM ANSWER SHEET

1. Ⓐ Ⓑ Ⓒ Ⓓ
2. Ⓐ Ⓑ Ⓒ Ⓓ
3. Ⓐ Ⓑ Ⓒ Ⓓ
4. Ⓐ Ⓑ Ⓒ Ⓓ
5. Ⓐ Ⓑ Ⓒ Ⓓ
6. Ⓐ Ⓑ Ⓒ Ⓓ
7. Ⓐ Ⓑ Ⓒ Ⓓ
8. Ⓐ Ⓑ Ⓒ Ⓓ
9. Ⓐ Ⓑ Ⓒ Ⓓ
10. Ⓐ Ⓑ Ⓒ Ⓓ
11. Ⓐ Ⓑ Ⓒ Ⓓ
12. Ⓐ Ⓑ Ⓒ Ⓓ
13. Ⓐ Ⓑ Ⓒ Ⓓ
14. Ⓐ Ⓑ Ⓒ Ⓓ
15. Ⓐ Ⓑ Ⓒ Ⓓ

16. Ⓐ Ⓑ Ⓒ Ⓓ
17. Ⓐ Ⓑ Ⓒ Ⓓ
18. Ⓐ Ⓑ Ⓒ Ⓓ
19. Ⓐ Ⓑ Ⓒ Ⓓ
20. Ⓐ Ⓑ Ⓒ Ⓓ
21. Ⓐ Ⓑ Ⓒ Ⓓ
22. Ⓐ Ⓑ Ⓒ Ⓓ
23. Ⓐ Ⓑ Ⓒ Ⓓ
24. Ⓐ Ⓑ Ⓒ Ⓓ
25. Ⓐ Ⓑ Ⓒ Ⓓ
26. Ⓐ Ⓑ Ⓒ Ⓓ
27. Ⓐ Ⓑ Ⓒ Ⓓ
28. Ⓐ Ⓑ Ⓒ Ⓓ
29. Ⓐ Ⓑ Ⓒ Ⓓ
30. Ⓐ Ⓑ Ⓒ Ⓓ

31. Ⓐ Ⓑ Ⓒ Ⓓ
32. Ⓐ Ⓑ Ⓒ Ⓓ
33. Ⓐ Ⓑ Ⓒ Ⓓ
34. Ⓐ Ⓑ Ⓒ Ⓓ
35. Ⓐ Ⓑ Ⓒ Ⓓ
36. Ⓐ Ⓑ Ⓒ Ⓓ
37. Ⓐ Ⓑ Ⓒ Ⓓ
38. Ⓐ Ⓑ Ⓒ Ⓓ
39. Ⓐ Ⓑ Ⓒ Ⓓ
40. Ⓐ Ⓑ Ⓒ Ⓓ
41. Ⓐ Ⓑ Ⓒ Ⓓ
42. Ⓐ Ⓑ Ⓒ Ⓓ
43. Ⓐ Ⓑ Ⓒ Ⓓ
44. Ⓐ Ⓑ Ⓒ Ⓓ
45. Ⓐ Ⓑ Ⓒ Ⓓ

46. Ⓐ Ⓑ Ⓒ Ⓓ
47. Ⓐ Ⓑ Ⓒ Ⓓ
48. Ⓐ Ⓑ Ⓒ Ⓓ
49. Ⓐ Ⓑ Ⓒ Ⓓ
50. Ⓐ Ⓑ Ⓒ Ⓓ
51. Ⓐ Ⓑ Ⓒ Ⓓ
52. Ⓐ Ⓑ Ⓒ Ⓓ
53. Ⓐ Ⓑ Ⓒ Ⓓ
54. Ⓐ Ⓑ Ⓒ Ⓓ
55. Ⓐ Ⓑ Ⓒ Ⓓ
56. Ⓐ Ⓑ Ⓒ Ⓓ
57. Ⓐ Ⓑ Ⓒ Ⓓ
58. Ⓐ Ⓑ Ⓒ Ⓓ
59. Ⓐ Ⓑ Ⓒ Ⓓ
60. Ⓐ Ⓑ Ⓒ Ⓓ

PRACTICE TEST 1: CNA/HHA EXAM

90 minutes—60 questions

> **Directions:** Read each question below and choose the correct answer from the four choices provided. Only one choice is correct, so choose carefully.

1. After reviewing data of a patient admitted to a psychiatric unit, the concern that has priority is the report of

    A. family trouble.

    B. suicidal thoughts.

    C. physical abuse.

    D. depression.

2. If patients are experiencing emesis in the bathroom, then they are

    A. defecating.

    B. vomiting.

    C. using the urinal.

    D. maintaining equal input and output.

3. A person who suffers from anxiety disorders should refrain from all of these EXCEPT:

    A. Coffee

    B. Chocolate

    C. Alcohol

    D. Exercise

4. If a CNA sees a call light on for a resident that is assigned to another aide, the CNA should

    A. let the resident's aide know.

    B. answer it anyway.

    C. send someone who is available.

    D. ignore it until they have time to respond.

5. Occult blood in stool means that it is

    A. present.

    B. continuous.

    C. hidden.

    D. dark.

6. While making rounds, the nursing assistant finds a patient on the floor. What is the first necessary step?

    A. Perform CPR.

    B. Call 911.

    C. Call the head nurse.

    D. Check for the patient's pulse and respiration.

7. If a patient is having breakfast and their hand is at their throat, the first thing to do is

    A. treat the patient with the Heimlich maneuver.

    B. hit the patient's back.

    C. give the patient water.

    D. ask the patient if they are choking.

8. The healthcare of the elderly is called

    A. genitourinary.

    B. geriatrics.

    C. pediatrics.

    D. genetics.

9. A Hindu patient refuses to take a prescribed medication from a gelatin capsule because it may contain

    A. vegetable filler.

    B. dairy filler.

    C. beef and pork fat.

    D. fruit filler.

10. The most effective way to minimize the spread of infection is by

    A. using a hand sanitizer.

    B. wearing masks.

    C. standing six feet apart.

    D. handwashing.

11. If a patient requires a medication twice per day, then the chart will state

    A. B/P.

    B. B.I.D.

    C. BM.

    D. BSC.

12. A susceptible host for infection means that a person

    A. has a disease.

    B. has poor immunity or low resistance.

    C. is in the best health.

    D. can fight off an infection.

13. Being accountable for providing care according to a recognized standard is the legal term for

    A. liability.

    B. aiding and abetting.

    C. ethics.

    D. passive neglect.

14. When documenting in a patient's record, it is necessary to perform all of these steps EXCEPT:

    A. Writing the date in the record

    B. Signing the record

    C. Spell-checking the record

    D. Writing in pencil so you can easily keep the record neat

15. An activity of daily living that is helpful to the entire body to prevent muscle atrophy is

    A. eating.

    B. taking vitamins.

    C. exercise.

    D. sleeping.

16. When helping a recovering stroke patient who has damage to the left side of their brain get dressed in a shirt, assistance should be given

    A. on the left side.

    B. behind the patient.

    C. on the right side.

    D. in front of the patient.

17. After checking all vitals on a patient, the reading that should be reported STAT is a

    A. radial pulse of 90 bpm.

    B. blood pressure reading of 200/100 mm Hg.

    C. respiration rate of 16 bpm.

    D. temperature reading of 99.9°.

18. The federal agency that sets and enforces workplace safety and health standards is

    A. Occupational Safety and Health Administration (OSHA).

    B. Material Safety Data Sheet (MSDS).

    C. Centers for Disease Control (CDC).

    D. National Institutes of Health (NIH).

19. When helping to move a patient from bed to chair, most of the patient's weight should be supported by the aide's

    A. back.

    B. legs.

    C. hips.

    D. arms.

20. Typically, if an aide is interested in and paying close attention to a conversation with the patient, they will

    A. lean forward.

    B. clasp hands.

    C. cross arms.

    D. slouch.

21. If a patient must have their leg joints stretched by the CNA while exercising, the patient is performing a

    A. passive ROM exercise.

    B. pivot.

    C. supine position.

    D. C diff.

22. A useful technique to encourage a patient to talk about how they are feeling is

    A. listening.

    B. asking open-ended questions.

    C. using body language.

    D. making jokes.

23. Before transporting a patient in a wheelchair through an open door, a CNA should check

    A. for traffic.

    B. the wheelchair's foot pedals.

    C. that the patient is secure.

    D. that the patient is comfortable.

24. The dirtiest part of the body is/are the

    A. rectum.

    B. armpits.

    C. mouth.

    D. hands.

25. *Candida Albicans* is commonly known as

    A. the flu.

    B. a yeast infection.

    C. a cold.

    D. an ear infection.

26. Patients who hear voices or see things that are not there are known to be

    A. depressed.

    B. hallucinating.

    C. manic.

    D. obsessive compulsive.

27. The permission granted by a patient after understanding the risks, benefits, and alternatives to a procedure or treatment plan is

    A. confidentiality.

    B. signed consent.

    C. informed consent.

    D. informed permission.

28. After a surgery, an aide sees NPO written in a patient's chart and knows the patient

    A. is experiencing nausea and vomiting.

    B. has no known allergies.

    C. cannot receive any foods or liquids by mouth.

    D. is hard of hearing.

29. When a patient leaves a hospital intentionally and without permission, it is considered an

    A. incident.

    B. identification.

    C. elopement.

    D. accident.

30. A temperature that is higher than what is within the normal range is a

    A. fever.

    B. shiver.

    C. sweat.

    D. chill.

31. When a CNA is tending to a patient who is using a restraint, the aide should

    A. release the restraint twice per shift.

    B. observe the patient every hour.

    C. make certain the restraint is loose.

    D. ensure the patient's body alignment is correct.

32. The science that explores how the body uses food is

   A. health.

   B. biology.

   C. physics.

   D. nutrition.

33. Static posture is

   A. how a person holds their body when they are moving.

   B. abnormal inward curving of the spine.

   C. how a person holds their body when they are not moving.

   D. rounded shoulders giving an individual excessive back curve.

34. A patient who has a false belief that clashes with reality is known to suffer from

   A. insomnia.

   B. agitation.

   C. delusion.

   D. depression.

35. In case of an emergency, the plan used to relocate patients to a safer location is called

   A. a fire drill.

   B. wandering.

   C. pacing.

   D. an evacuation plan.

36. When a patient's movement or behavior is limited in a physical or chemical way, they are

   A. restrained.

   B. disoriented.

   C. paralyzed.

   D. asleep.

37. To prevent pulling on a male patient's catheter tube when turning him, an aide should tape the tube to

   A. his abdomen.

   B. his hip.

   C. his upper thigh.

   D. the bed rail.

38. The community that offers some support but not a high level of care is a(n)_____ facility.

   A. nursing home

   B. independent living

   C. assisted living

   D. leisure

39. The key element needed for microbe growth is

   A. salt.

   B. extreme heat.

   C. extreme cold.

   D. moisture.

40. When a resident with a speech impairment is having a difficult time communicating, try to AVOID

   A. trying to complete their sentences.

   B. taking the time to listen.

   C. allowing a pause in the conversation.

   D. using pen and paper to write any words they are having a hard time communicating.

41. A computer information system that stores and saves a patient's medical data is a(n)

   A. chart.

   B. electronic health record.

   C. filing cabinet.

D. off-site storage facility.

42. Basic rules between patients, healthcare providers, and the organizations that support them are _____ rights.

    A. human

    B. patient

    C. civil

    D. privacy

43. In watching a patient move to the bed, an aide notices a spill on the floor and must

    A. put up a caution cone.

    B. quickly clean it up.

    C. call housekeeping.

    D. call another aide to assist.

44. Hypertension is more commonly referred to as high

    A. blood sugar.

    B. cholesterol.

    C. blood pressure.

    D. blood platelets.

45. Supination is turning a body part

    A. inward.

    B. outward.

    C. downward.

    D. upward.

46. As the patient and his family are ready to pray before their meal, a nursing assistant should NOT

    A. give them privacy.

    B. tell them they cannot pray outside their room.

    C. excuse themself and wait outside the door.

D. ask them if they need anything before excusing themself.

47. All of these are common types of microorganisms EXCEPT:

    A. Bacteria

    B. Viruses

    C. Protozoa

    D. Toxins

48. While pushing a very anxious patient in their wheelchair during the start of a fire alarm, the CNA should

    A. calm the patient and then leave to search for assistance.

    B. lock the wheelchair and leave the area to check for smoke.

    C. move the wheelchair and carry the patient out of the facility.

    D. calm the patient while moving them to a safe place.

49. Anything that can cause harm to the safety of a patient is a(n)

    A. hazard.

    B. disaster.

    C. prevention.

    D. awareness.

50. Physicians that deal with mental health issues and can write prescriptions are

    A. psychiatrists.

    B. psychologists.

C. counselors.

D. therapists.

51. The interdisciplinary care plan communicates the

    A. goals and treatment plans for the patients ordered by the physician.

    B. needs of the patient and creates practices to meet those needs by the healthcare team.

    C. specific plan of care for each patient developed by the nursing team.

    D. needs of the financial plan for each patient.

52. Which is NOT considered a range of motion exercise?

    A. Passive active

    B. Active

    C. Active assisted

    D. Passive

53. Allowing a patient to talk about their cultural and spiritual beliefs does not have an impact on

    A. the quality of care they receive.

    B. their mental health.

    C. their physical health.

    D. their ability to connect with their caregiver.

54. To prevent the spread of infection in a facility, it is important to do all of these EXCEPT:

    A. Wash hands only at the start of a shift

    B. Dispose of dirty supplies

    C. Keep a clean environment

    D. Wear necessary gear

55. The pedal pulse is on the

    A. elbow.

    B. foot.

C. wrist.

D. neck.

56. A complaint or objection filed by a patient about their care or living space is

    A. a grievance.

    B. defamation of character.

    C. a violation.

    D. coercion.

57. Which of the following can help guard a person from falling off the bed when sleeping?

    A. Restraint

    B. Cane

    C. Bedrail

    D. Walker

58. While they are in conversation, the CNA can let the patient know they are listening by

    A. turning in the patient's direction while working.

    B. turning in the patient's direction and answering when appropriate.

    C. talking about family life to engage the patient.

    D. asking more questions to direct the conversation.

59. Claustrophobia is the extreme fear of

    A. blood.

    B. heights.

    C. open spaces.

    D. crowded or cramped spaces.

60. A hospital's procedure to react safely and correctly to a fire is to follow

    A. P.P.E.

    B. R.A.C.E.

    C. P.A.S.S.

    D. M.S.D.S.

ANSWER KEY AND EXPLANATIONS

1. B	11. B	21. A	31. D	41. B	51. B
2. B	12. B	22. B	32. D	42. B	52. A
3. D	13. A	23. A	33. C	43. B	53. A
4. B	14. D	24. C	34. C	44. C	54. A
5. C	15. C	25. B	35. D	45. D	55. B
6. D	16. C	26. B	36. A	46. B	56. A
7. D	17. B	27. C	37. C	47. D	57. C
8. B	18. A	28. C	38. C	48. D	58. B
9. C	19. B	29. C	39. D	49. A	59. D
10. D	20. A	30. A	40. A	50. A	60. B

1. **The correct answer is B.** Reports of suicidal thoughts always have top priority for patients admitted to the psychiatric unit. Reports of family trouble (choice A), reports of physical abuse (choice C), and reports of depression (choice D) are also important but do not have top priority.

2. **The correct answer is B.** Patients who experience emesis are vomiting. Having a bowel movement is defecating (choice A). A urinal (choice C) is a bottle used for urination. Fluid balance is maintaining equal input and output (choice D).

3. **The correct answer is D.** Exercise provides the body with natural calming chemicals, endorphins, which help to relieve anxiety. Coffee (choice A), chocolate (choice B), and alcohol (choice C) can increase anxiety.

4. **The correct answer is B.** Even if an aide must step in for another co-worker, it is important to answer the call light anyway and provide patient care. After checking in on the patient, let the resident aide know what the issue is so they can respond to it (choice A). Sending someone who is available (choice C) may take additional time, so answering the call light immediately is the most efficient response. Ignoring it until you have a minute (choice D) may have negative consequences, especially if the resident is experiencing an emergency.

5. **The correct answer is C.** Occult blood in stool means that it is hidden from view. Occult blood can be present (choice A), continuous (choice B), and dark (choice D) but cannot be seen.

6. **The correct answer is D.** Since the patient could have fainted, establishing a pulse and a respiration rate are the first functions the nursing assistant is required to check. Therefore, performing CPR (choice A), calling 911 (choice B), and calling the head nurse (choice C) are not the first actions to carry out.

7. **The correct answer is D.** It is always important to ask a patient if they are choking first. Treating the patient with the Heimlich maneuver (choice A), hitting the patient's back (choice B), or giving the patient water (choice C) are options to help them only after knowing if the patient is choking first.

8. **The correct answer is B.** Geriatrics is the area of medicine that deals with the healthcare of the elderly. Genitourinary (choice A) are the functions and organs of the urine and genital systems. Pediatrics (choice C) is the healthcare of children. Genetics (choice D) is the area of science that deals with the study of genes.

9. **The correct answer is C.** Since the gelatin in the capsule may be made from beef or pork and Hindus believe in reincarnation of all living creatures, a patient may refuse to take the medication.

Taking medication with gelatin containing a vegetable filler (choice A), a dairy filler (choice B), and a fruit filler (choice D) would not go against their beliefs.

10. **The correct answer is D.** Handwashing is the most effective way to minimize the spread of infection. Using a hand sanitizer (choice A), wearing masks (choice B), and standing six feet apart (choice C) can help minimize the spread of infections but are not the most effective methods.

11. **The correct answer is B.** A chart with B.I.D. written means that the patient is taking the medication twice daily. B/P (choice A) indicates blood pressure measurement. BM (choice C) indicates a bowel movement. BSC (choice D) indicates a patient has a bedside commode.

12. **The correct answer is B.** A person who has poor immunity or low resistance is a susceptible host for disease or infection. A person who has an infection (choice A) is no longer susceptible. A person who is in the best health (choice C) has the greatest opportunity to fight off an infection (choice D).

13. **The correct answer is A.** Liability is the legal term used for being accountable for providing care according to a recognized standard. Aiding and abetting is someone who assists or encourages someone in a crime (choice B). Ethics (choice C) are moral beliefs that govern someone's behavior. Inadvertently harming a patient physically, mentally, or emotionally by failing to provide needed care is passive neglect (choice D).

14. **The correct answer is D.** Since the record is a legal document, writing in pencil, where information could be easily altered, is not an option. Writing the date in the record (choice A), signing the record (choice B), and spell-checking the record (choice C) are all steps to the process of documenting a patient's record.

15. **The correct answer is C.** Exercise keeps the body physically active and prevents atrophy of the muscles. Eating (choice A), taking vitamins (choice B), and sleeping (choice C) are all necessary for the body but do not prevent muscle atrophy.

16. **The correct answer is C.** Assistance should begin on the right side since that is where the patient is weakest and will best allow balance support. Starting on the left side (choice A), behind the patient (choice B), and in front of the patient (choice D) does not offer the best balanced support for dressing.

17. **The correct answer is B.** Normal blood pressure is 120/80 mm Hg, so a high blood pressure reading of 200/100 mm Hg should be reported immediately. A radial pulse of 90 bpm (choice A) and a respiration rate of 16 bpm (choice D) both fall within normal limits. A temperature reading of 100.0° (choice D) is considered a low-grade fever, but not required to be labeled as STAT.

18. **The correct answer is A.** The federal agency that sets and enforces workplace safety and health standards is OSHA. The MSDS (choice B) is the document that handles information, response, and handling of dangerous chemicals in the workplace. The CDC (choice C) handles the health surveillance of disease outbreak and health statistics. The NIH (choice D) is the world's organizational leader in medical research.

19. **The correct answer is B.** After assessing a patient's ability to help with the move, an aide should use their legs to bare most of the patient's weight. To avoid undue stress and minimize injury to an aide's body, it is best not to use the back (choice A), the hips (choice C), or the arms (choice D) as the primary sources for bearing a patient's weight.

20. **The correct answer is A.** Leaning forward during a conversation will help an aide to build rapport with the resident. Clasped hands (choice B), crossing arms (choice C) and slouching (choice D) are closed postures that communicate unpleasant feelings.

21. **The correct answer is A.** Passive range of motion exercises are completed by the CNA with little to no assistance from the patient. Pivot (choice A) is a point on which something turns or hinges. Supine position (choice C) is when a patient is lying face up on their back. C diff (choice D) is a bacterium

that causes diarrhea and inflammation of the colon.

22. **The correct answer is B.** Asking open-ended questions allows a patient to talk rather than answer in a "yes" or "no" format. Listening (choice A) and using body language (choice C) do not use verbal communication. Making jokes (choice D) can make a patient feel uncomfortable and discourage speech.

23. **The correct answer is A.** Before going through an open door with a patient in a wheelchair, always check for traffic coming in all directions. Checking the foot pedals (choice A), checking to be sure the patient is secure (choice C), and checking to be sure the patient is comfortable (choice D) should be verified prior to transporting them anywhere.

24. **The correct answer is C.** The mouth is the dirtiest part of the body because it has the largest number of bacteria. The rectum (choice A) has the second largest number of bacteria. Although having a great deal of bacteria, the armpits (choice B) and the hands (choice D) are not the dirtiest parts of the body.

25. **The correct answer is B.** A yeast infection comes from the fungus, *Candida Albicans*. The flu (choice A), a cold (choice C), and an ear infection (choice D) come from different bacteria and/or viruses.

26. **The correct answer is B.** Hallucinations are events that occur through all five senses but are not real. Depression (choice A) is a constant state of feeling sad. A manic (choice C) patient experiences an intense euphoric mood or has extreme energy. Obsessive compulsive (choice D) patients have uncontrollable and repetitive thoughts and behaviors.

27. **The correct answer is C.** Patients that give informed consent understand the risks, benefits and alternatives involved in a procedure or treatment plan. Confidentiality (choice A) is applied by not releasing private information to anyone who should not or does not need to know about a patient. Signed consent (choice B) and informed

permission (choice D) are not legally valid consent options.

28. **The correct answer is C.** If NPO is written in a patient's chart after surgery, they cannot receive any foods or liquids by mouth. If a patient is experiencing nausea and vomiting (choice A), a nurse's aide will see n/v written in their chart. If a patient has NKA written in their chart, then the patient has no known allergies (choice B). If a patient has HOH written in their chart, then the patient is hard of hearing (choice D).

29. **The correct answer is C.** An elopement is when a patient leaves a facility against medical advice. An incident (choice A) is a situation that can harm a patient or any other person. An identification (choice B) is a patient's sense of identity. An accident (choice D) is an unplanned event or situation.

30. **The correct answer is A.** A fever is a temperature higher than what is considered the normal range. A shiver (choice B), sweat (choice C), and chill (choice D) are all symptoms of a fever.

31. **The correct answer is D.** If a patient is required to have restraints, it is necessary for the staff to follow the strict practices in the physician's orders to maintain their safety. In keeping in line with the facility's policies for patient restraints, releasing the restraint twice per shift (choice A), observing the patient every hour (choice B), and making certain the restraint is loose (choice C) will need to be specified and documented by the physician.

32. **The correct answer is D.** Nutrition is the science that studies how the body uses food. Health (choice A) is the condition of being well physically, mentally, and emotionally. Biology (choice B) is the study of life. Physics (choice C) is the science that studies the interactions of matter and energy.

33. **The correct answer is C.** Sitting, standing, and sleeping are forms of static posture. Dynamic posture is how a person holds their body when they are moving (choice A). Lordosis is the abnormal inward curving of the spine (choice B). Kyphosis posture is having rounded shoulders, giving a person an excessive back curve (choice D).

34. **The correct answer is C.** A patient who suffers from delusions has views or beliefs that conflict with reality. Insomnia (choice A) is the inability to sleep. Agitation (choice B) is the feeling of being restless and irritated. Depression (choice D) is a constant state of feeling sad.

35. **The correct answer is D.** An evacuation plan allows patients to be safely relocated during an emergency. A fire drill (choice A) is practicing a plan to ensure proper evacuation of people in case of a fire. Wandering (choice B) is aimless walking throughout a facility. Pacing (choice C) is walking back and forth consistently in the same place.

36. **The correct answer is A.** When they are a danger to themselves or others, a patient's movement or behavior is restrained in a physical or chemical way. A patient can become disoriented (choice B) about a person, place, or time. If a patient is paralyzed (choice C), then they have lost muscle and bodily functions. When a patient is asleep (choice D), their movements and behaviors are not limited.

37. **The correct answer is C.** An indwelling catheter tube cannot be kinked or pulled and needs to be taped or specially fastened to the patient's upper thigh. Since the drainage bag needs to be lower than the patient's bladder, taping the catheter tube to the abdomen (choice A), hip (choice B), and the bed rail (choice D) can cause a backflow of urine.

38. **The correct answer is C.** Assisted living facilities offer care that is designed for senior citizens who need some support with daily activities but do not need care in a nursing home. A nursing home facility (choice A) is a place where people do not need to be in a hospital but cannot be cared for at home. An independent living facility (choice B) is designed for older people who want the convenience of easier living but do not require any assistance. A leisure facility (choice D) is designed to provide high-level activities for older people.

39. **The correct answer is D.** Moisture is the key element for microbe growth. Salt (choice A), extreme heat (choice B), and extreme cold (choice C) limit microbe growth.

40. **The correct answer is A.** Completing the sentence of a patient with a speech impairment can be frustrating and make them feel rushed. Taking the time to listen (choice B), allowing a pause in the conversation to let them work through it (choice C), and using pen and paper to write any words they are having a hard time communicating (choice D) are ways to help a resident with a speech impairment convey their message.

41. **The correct answer is B.** An electronic health record allows the patient's medical data to be stored and saved via a computer information system. A chart (choice A) stores and saves the patient's written medical data on paper. A filing cabinet (choice C) and an off-site storage facility (choice D) are ways to physically store and save patient's written medical data.

42. **The correct answer is B.** Patient rights are federal and state laws that guarantee patients certain established rights in the health care system between providers, patients, and the organizations that support them. Human rights (choice A) are basic rights and freedoms given to all people. Civil rights (choice C) are given based on an agreement between the citizen and the country or state in which the citizen resides. Privacy rights (choice D) are the idea that an individual's personal information is protected from public examination.

43. **The correct answer is B.** Since falls can lead to injuries, it is important to quickly clean up a spill. It is necessary not to overlook a possible cause of a fall by putting up a caution cone (choice A). Since it is essential for staff to continuously be on alert for possible hazards, calling housekeeping (choice C) and calling another aide to assist (choice D) only delays a quick response.

44. **The correct answer is C.** High blood pressure is the common name for hypertension. High blood sugar (choice A) is known as hyperglycemia. High cholesterol (choice B) is known as hyperlipidemia. Having high platelets (choice D) is called thrombocytosis.

45. **The correct answer is D.** Turning a body part upward is supination. Inversion is turning a body

part inward (choice A). Turning a body part outward is eversion (choice B). Pronation is turning a body part downward (choice C).

46. **The correct answer is B.** To be within their rights to express their beliefs, a patient should not be told they cannot pray outside their room. Patients should be given privacy (choice A) should they want it. Nursing assistants can respectfully excuse themselves and wait outside the door (choice C) while the patient prays, and they can ask the patient if they need anything before excusing themselves (choice D).

47. **The correct answer is D.** Since toxins are a poisonous substance, they are not microorganisms. Bacteria (choice A), viruses (choice B), and protozoa (choice C) are all microorganisms.

48. **The correct answer is D.** Since the CNA is responsible for knowing fire safety policies and procedures, calming the patient and moving them to a safe place is protocol. Calming the patient and then leaving to search for assistance (choice A), locking the wheelchair and leaving the area to check for smoke (choice B), and moving the wheelchair to carry the patient out of the facility (choice C) are not the correct techniques to use to respond to the fire safety protocols put in place by the facility.

49. **The correct answer is A.** A hazard is something in a patient's setting that can cause harm to their safety. A disaster (choice B) is a sudden catastrophic event that can bring harm to a patient or property. Prevention (choice C) is the attempt to stop something from happening. Awareness (choice D) is knowing a fact about a situation.

50. **The correct answer is A.** Psychiatrists are physicians who deal with mental health issues and can write prescriptions. Although psychologists (choice B), counselors (choice C), and therapists (choice D) can provide mental health services, they cannot write prescriptions for medications.

51. **The correct answer is B.** The interdisciplinary care plan determines the needs of the patient and creates practices to meet those needs. The goals and treatment plans for the patients ordered by the physician are an aspect of the interdisciplinary care plan (choice A). The specific plan of care for each patient that is developed by the nursing team (choice C) is developed from the interdisciplinary care plan. The financial plan for each patient (choice D) is an aspect of the interdisciplinary care plan.

52. **The correct answer is A.** There are either passive or active range of motion exercises, but not passive active. Active (choice B) range of motion exercise is done by the patient with no assistance. Active assisted (choice C) range of motion exercise is done by the patient with some assistance by another person or machine. Passive (choice D) range of motion exercise is not done by the patient at all but done completely by another person or machine.

53. **The correct answer is A.** A patient's cultural and spiritual beliefs should never impact the quality of care they receive. Allowing a patient to talk about their cultural and spiritual beliefs typically has a positive impact on their mental health (choice B), their physical health (choice C), and their ability to connect with their caregiver (choice D).

54. **The correct answer is A.** Preventing the spread of infection requires constant handwashing, not just at the start of a shift. Disposing of dirty supplies (choice B), keeping a clean environment (choice C), and wearing necessary gear (choice D) are all ways to prevent the spread of infection.

55. **The correct answer is B.** The pedal pulse is on the top of the foot. Brachial pulse is at the elbow (choice A). Radial pulse is at the wrist (choice C). Carotid pulse is at the neck (choice D).

56. **The correct answer is A.** A grievance is a formal complaint filed by a patient about their care or living space. Defamation (choice B) is communication that is not true and harms someone's good name or reputation. A violation (choice C) is a breach or an infringement. Coercion (choice D) is forcing someone to do something against their will.

57. **The correct answer is C.** The bedrail serves as a guard to help prevent someone from falling off a bed. A restraint (choice A) is a device used to limit a patient's movement. Canes (choice B) and walkers (choice D) are devices used to help patients with balance while walking.

58. **The correct answer is B.** To let the patient know the CNA is engaged in the conversation and what the patient is saying is important, it is necessary to turn in the patient's direction and answer when appropriate. Turning in the patient's direction while working (choice A), talking about family life to engage the patient (choice C), and asking more questions as to direct the conversation (choice D) may discourage the patient from having more conversation in the future.

59. **The correct answer is D.** The extreme fear of cramped or crowded spaces is claustrophobia. Hemophobia (choice A) is the extreme fear of blood. Acrophobia (choice B) is the extreme fear of heights. Agoraphobia (choice C) is the extreme fear of open spaces.

60. **The correct answer is B.** R.A.C.E (Remove, Activate, Contain, Extinguish) is the hospital's procedure to react safely and correctly to a fire. Personal Protective Equipment, P.P.E. (choice A), is equipment worn by medical staff to reduce the risk of spreading germs. Pull, Aim, Squeeze, and Sweep or P.A.S.S. (choice C) is the technique used to handle a fire extinguisher. The MSDS (choice D) is the document that handles information, response, and handling of dangerous chemicals in the workplace.

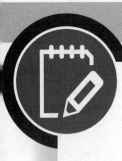

NOTES

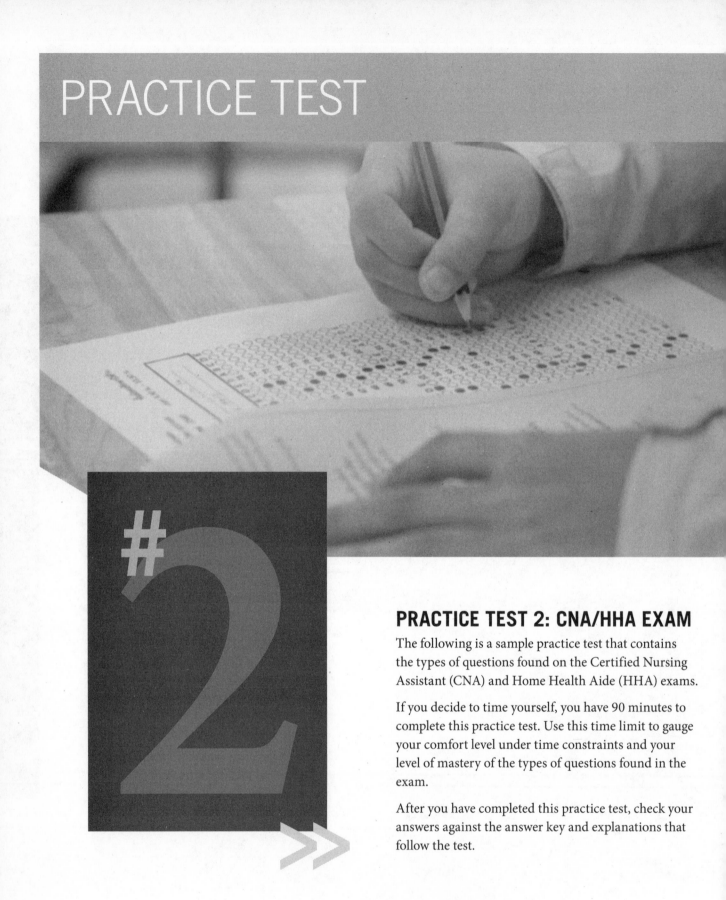

PRACTICE TEST

PRACTICE TEST 2: CNA/HHA EXAM

The following is a sample practice test that contains the types of questions found on the Certified Nursing Assistant (CNA) and Home Health Aide (HHA) exams.

If you decide to time yourself, you have 90 minutes to complete this practice test. Use this time limit to gauge your comfort level under time constraints and your level of mastery of the types of questions found in the exam.

After you have completed this practice test, check your answers against the answer key and explanations that follow the test.

PRACTICE TEST 2: CNA/HHA EXAM ANSWER SHEET

1. Ⓐ Ⓑ Ⓒ Ⓓ   16. Ⓐ Ⓑ Ⓒ Ⓓ   31. Ⓐ Ⓑ Ⓒ Ⓓ   46. Ⓐ Ⓑ Ⓒ Ⓓ

2. Ⓐ Ⓑ Ⓒ Ⓓ   17. Ⓐ Ⓑ Ⓒ Ⓓ   32. Ⓐ Ⓑ Ⓒ Ⓓ   47. Ⓐ Ⓑ Ⓒ Ⓓ

3. Ⓐ Ⓑ Ⓒ Ⓓ   18. Ⓐ Ⓑ Ⓒ Ⓓ   33. Ⓐ Ⓑ Ⓒ Ⓓ   48. Ⓐ Ⓑ Ⓒ Ⓓ

4. Ⓐ Ⓑ Ⓒ Ⓓ   19. Ⓐ Ⓑ Ⓒ Ⓓ   34. Ⓐ Ⓑ Ⓒ Ⓓ   49. Ⓐ Ⓑ Ⓒ Ⓓ

5. Ⓐ Ⓑ Ⓒ Ⓓ   20. Ⓐ Ⓑ Ⓒ Ⓓ   35. Ⓐ Ⓑ Ⓒ Ⓓ   50. Ⓐ Ⓑ Ⓒ Ⓓ

6. Ⓐ Ⓑ Ⓒ Ⓓ   21. Ⓐ Ⓑ Ⓒ Ⓓ   36. Ⓐ Ⓑ Ⓒ Ⓓ   51. Ⓐ Ⓑ Ⓒ Ⓓ

7. Ⓐ Ⓑ Ⓒ Ⓓ   22. Ⓐ Ⓑ Ⓒ Ⓓ   37. Ⓐ Ⓑ Ⓒ Ⓓ   52. Ⓐ Ⓑ Ⓒ Ⓓ

8. Ⓐ Ⓑ Ⓒ Ⓓ   23. Ⓐ Ⓑ Ⓒ Ⓓ   38. Ⓐ Ⓑ Ⓒ Ⓓ   53. Ⓐ Ⓑ Ⓒ Ⓓ

9. Ⓐ Ⓑ Ⓒ Ⓓ   24. Ⓐ Ⓑ Ⓒ Ⓓ   39. Ⓐ Ⓑ Ⓒ Ⓓ   54. Ⓐ Ⓑ Ⓒ Ⓓ

10. Ⓐ Ⓑ Ⓒ Ⓓ   25. Ⓐ Ⓑ Ⓒ Ⓓ   40. Ⓐ Ⓑ Ⓒ Ⓓ   55. Ⓐ Ⓑ Ⓒ Ⓓ

11. Ⓐ Ⓑ Ⓒ Ⓓ   26. Ⓐ Ⓑ Ⓒ Ⓓ   41. Ⓐ Ⓑ Ⓒ Ⓓ   56. Ⓐ Ⓑ Ⓒ Ⓓ

12. Ⓐ Ⓑ Ⓒ Ⓓ   27. Ⓐ Ⓑ Ⓒ Ⓓ   42. Ⓐ Ⓑ Ⓒ Ⓓ   57. Ⓐ Ⓑ Ⓒ Ⓓ

13. Ⓐ Ⓑ Ⓒ Ⓓ   28. Ⓐ Ⓑ Ⓒ Ⓓ   43. Ⓐ Ⓑ Ⓒ Ⓓ   58. Ⓐ Ⓑ Ⓒ Ⓓ

14. Ⓐ Ⓑ Ⓒ Ⓓ   29. Ⓐ Ⓑ Ⓒ Ⓓ   44. Ⓐ Ⓑ Ⓒ Ⓓ   59. Ⓐ Ⓑ Ⓒ Ⓓ

15. Ⓐ Ⓑ Ⓒ Ⓓ   30. Ⓐ Ⓑ Ⓒ Ⓓ   45. Ⓐ Ⓑ Ⓒ Ⓓ   60. Ⓐ Ⓑ Ⓒ Ⓓ

PRACTICE TEST 2: CNA/HHA EXAM

90 minutes—60 questions

> **Directions:** Read each question below and choose the correct answer from the four choices provided. Only one choice is correct, so choose carefully.

1. The nutritional guide that represents the standards of good nutrition is the
   A. DASH dietary guidelines.
   B. food pyramid.
   C. National Health and Nutrition Examination Survey (NHANES).
   D. United States Department of Agriculture (USDA).

2. The right way to give abdominal thrusts during the Heimlich maneuver to a choking person is to
   A. push down while laying the hands flat on the abdomen.
   B. quickly push downward while pressing one fist against the abdomen.
   C. tenderly thrust downward with the fist.
   D. make a fist, place the thumb side against the abdomen, and rapidly thrust upward.

3. Excessive straightening of a body part is called
   A. flexion.
   B. extension.
   C. dorsiflexion.
   D. hyperextension.

4. When working with a manual bed, a CNA should always
   A. turn the cranks clockwise to lock the bed.
   B. turn the cranks counterclockwise to unlock the bed.
   C. elevate the patient's head.
   D. fold the cranks under the bed.

5. If a nurse's aide is trying to communicate with a completely deaf patient, the aide should
   A. project their voice as loud as possible.
   B. use a system of alarm rings.
   C. use a pen and paper or a typing device.
   D. use the Braille notation system.

6. If a physician is caring for a cardiology patient and is looking for a CBC, they are asking for the
   A. complete blood count.
   B. complete blood catheter.
   C. center for blood diseases.
   D. center for blood disorders.

7. A patient's dressing should always
   A. remain clean and dry.
   B. be allowed to air dry.
   C. be fastened by tape.
   D. be close-fitting to keep out bacteria.

8. The process of killing all harmful viruses and bacteria is called
   A. sanitation.
   B. clean technique.
   C. disinfection.
   D. handwashing.

9. A resident who has trouble recalling, learning new things, focusing, or making everyday life decisions has

   A. cognitive impairment.

   B. developmental disorders.

   C. motor skill disorders.

   D. Alzheimer's disease.

10. The written guidelines for the care of residents and the operation of a healthcare facility are

    A. the grievances.

    B. involuntary confinements.

    C. informed consents.

    D. its policies and procedures.

11. Which of the following provides the basic information about a person's bodily functions?

    A. Stethoscope

    B. Thermometer

    C. Otoscope

    D. Vital signs

12. The term used for "burping" and "passing gas" is

    A. fascia.

    B. flatus.

    C. fantod.

    D. facies.

13. The general term for the mental ability that declines and affects memory, reasoning, or other thinking skills is

    A. Alzheimer's disease.

    B. depression.

    C. bi-polar disorder.

    D. dementia.

14. The process of destroying all pathogens on medical instruments is called

    A. combustion.

    B. clean technique.

    C. autoclave.

    D. sterilization.

15. A patient wants to share a religious experience with a nursing assistant, so the assistant should

    A. sit and listen for as long as it takes.

    B. state that they are not allowed to discuss religion.

    C. listen and move on when the opportunity presents itself.

    D. tell this patient they are busy with another patient.

16. In a long-term care facility, if a patient with hepatitis accidentally steps on broken glass, the aide should

    A. call in the nurse to pick it up while they tend to the patient.

    B. call 911 and housekeeping.

    C. section off the area until it can be cleaned up.

    D. treat the patient at the site of the accident.

17. Rotating an upward-facing palm at the wrist until it faces the floor is an example of

    A. pronation.

    B. supination.

    C. rotation.

    D. opposition.

18. The minimum practices used to prevent infection, whether there is a confirmed or suspected case, are known as _____ precautions.

    A. contact

    B. standard

    C. transmission

    D. airborne

19. A common nosocomial infection is

    A. a urinary tract infection.

    B. shingles.

    C. human papilloma virus.

    D. chicken pox.

20. A defense mechanism used by elderly patients to relieve stress by returning to immature behavior is referred to as

    A. rationalization.

    B. projection.

    C. regression.

    D. repression.

21. A situation that causes serious illness and injury and needs a prompt response requires a

    A. patient to wait 24 hours.

    B. call to emergency medical services.

    C. visit to urgent care.

    D. visit to the primary care physician.

22. Many warning labels may consist of all of these EXCEPT:

    A. A local emergency system phone number

    B. Health and physical hazards

    C. Protective gear to wear

    D. Storage and disposal information

23. To effectively minimize the spread of germs, CNAs and HHAs should wash hands for at least

    A. 30 seconds.

    B. 10 seconds.

    C. 20 seconds.

    D. 60 seconds.

24. If a patient must take a medication only as needed and not scheduled, then it will be documented as

    A. QD.

    B. BID.

    C. PRN.

    D. TID.

25. If a patient with Alzheimer's disease is trying to communicate their needs, they may become agitated because they are all of these EXCEPT:

    A. Coping

    B. Disoriented

    C. Confused

    D. Combative

26. A DNR order has been placed in a patient's file to indicate that the patient is/has

    A. a fall risk.

    B. no brain function.

    C. not to be revived if the heart stops.

    D. to be revived.

27. The number of breaths taken per minute is measured as the

    A. respiratory rate.

    B. metabolic rate.

    C. heart rate.

    D. mortality rate.

28. Addiction changes

    A. only the behavior of the addict.

    B. only the physical appearance of the addict.

    C. the addict's brain chemistry.

    D. no one.

29. Failure to take responsibility, violation of others' rights, and lacking remorse are all signs of _____ personality disorder.

    A. antisocial

    B. borderline

    C. histrionic

    D. schizotypal

30. A nurse's aide is stuck by a sharp needle that was disposed of in the wrong container. The aide should immediately

    A. report it to the head nurse.

    B. try to pinch the blood out.

    C. wash the area for a few minutes.

    D. apply hand sanitizer and ointment.

31. Every time an aide washes hands, the soap should be applied

    A. before wetting the hands.

    B. before setting water temperature.

    C. after taking off the gloves.

    D. after wetting hands.

32. The inability to move the bottom half of the body is called

    A. cardioplegia.

    B. hemiplegia.

    C. paraplegia.

    D. quadriplegia.

33. Most conflicts for a resident arise from all of these EXCEPT:

    A. Poor communication

    B. Feeling misunderstood

    C. Making assumptions

    D. Listening

34. To accurately identify a new patient when entering the hospital room, the provider should first

    A. ask the family member in the room.

    B. wait for the nurse.

    C. look at the ID bracelet.

    D. treat them.

35. A document required to be completed after a fall or injury event that occurs to any person in a facility is a(n)

    A. risk management report.

    B. incident report.

    C. audit report.

    D. prevention assessment.

36. Since the aide notices that the patient begins her bath by cleaning her rectal area and then placing the washcloth back in the basin, the aide decides to

    A. clean the basin and replace the water.

    B. replace the washcloth.

    C. remind the patient that a bath begins with the face.

    D. continue with the bath after adding a disinfectant.

37. In understanding cultural practices, CNAs and HHAs should note that Americans view direct eye contact as

    A. rude, hostile, or sexually aggressive.

    B. disrespectful.

    C. a pathway to soul loss or theft.

    D. a way of showing honesty and candidness.

38. Cognition is

    A. the ability to apply knowledge.

    B. the mental activities involved in gaining knowledge and understanding.

    C. designed to assess your overall ability to solve problems and understand concepts.

    D. the science of how we think, learn, focus, solve problems, forget, and remember.

39. The most appropriate time to use a soft toothette for mouthcare is when a patient is

    A. wearing dentures.

    B. unconscious.

    C. complaining of a toothache.

    D. having a seizure.

40. To prevent the breakdown of skin, it is most important to

   A. fully dry the entire body.

   B. pat dry the body.

   C. apply lotion, especially between fingers and toes.

   D. air dry.

41. The purpose of log rolling is to

   A. keep the spine straight while turning or moving a patient.

   B. keep head and shoulders slightly elevated with a pillow.

   C. support the knee-elbow position with straps.

   D. keep the head of the patient's bed raised 30-90 degrees above the level and to sometimes elevate the knees.

42. All of these may occur if an aide decides not to use the prescribed gait belt to transfer a patient EXCEPT:

   A. Straining their back

   B. Shortening the process of the transfer

   C. Using more energy

   D. Having an increased risk of a patient falling

43. A form of non-verbal communication that can send a negative message to a patient is

   A. smiling.

   B. gently touching the shoulder.

   C. rolling the eyes.

   D. sarcastically responding.

44. All of these are commonly considered infectious EXCEPT:

   A. Plasma

   B. Tears

   C. Vaginal discharge

   D. Saliva

45. Patients who speak chaotically without a logical connection or lack relevance in conversation are

   A. tranquil.

   B. incoherent.

   C. vague.

   D. flat.

46. While taking vitals, the CNA notices a pressure sore has formed and calls the nurse to

   A. receive permission to dress the wound.

   B. have the patient move to a new position.

   C. dress the wound and assist in the process.

   D. have the nurse document the aide's observations.

47. The Health Insurance Portability and Account- ability Act (HIPAA) are federal laws which state that healthcare providers

   A. share patient health information with just the family.

   B. can only share appropriate patient information with those directly involved in caring for them.

   C. share patient health information with just the spouse.

   D. do not share patient health information with anyone.

48. When an elderly person is admitted to a long-term care facility, they have the right to

   A. possess personal items in the room.

   B. possess the items the facility says they can have.

   C. choose the items donated by the local thrift store.

   D. request specific items of their choosing to be paid for by the long-term facility.

49. Measuring temperature through the ear is referred to as _____ temperature.

   A. rectal

   B. tympanic

   C. temporal

   D. axillary

50. An example of positive body language is

   A. having eyes wide open with a smile.

   B. shrugging shoulders up.

   C. staring at a person with a puzzled look.

   D. nodding encouragingly as someone speaks.

51. The use of physical force to restrict freedom with or without a patient's consent is

   A. restraint.

   B. rationale for restraints.

   C. documentation of restraint.

   D. restraint assessment.

52. When feeding a quadriplegic, it is important to

   A. give small bites of food and permit enough time to chew.

   B. give fluids after the meal is done.

   C. rush through the meal.

   D. dress and groom the resident at the same time.

53. An important step to shaving a patient is to

   A. begin at the sideburns and shave sideways.

   B. shave downward on the neck.

   C. find out if the patient has a bleeding problem.

   D. have someone assist you.

54. The proper way to handle dirty linen is to

   A. wear gloves only when changing them.

   B. carry it away from the body.

   C. place it next to clean linen.

   D. dispose of it in the normal trash.

55. Cutting a resident's toenails is typically a responsibility given to a

   A. nursing assistant.

   B. family member.

   C. physical therapist.

   D. doctor or nurse.

56. If a patient has NPO written in their chart, then they

   A. cannot have anything by mouth.

   B. have a drug allergy.

   C. cannot eat solid food.

   D. have a food allergy.

57. Disinfection destroys

   A. just the nonpathogens.

   B. just the microbes.

   C. just the pathogens.

   D. all microbes, including the pathogens and nonpathogens.

58. A normal body temperature range is

   A. 95°-97° Fahrenheit.

   B. 100°-101° Fahrenheit.

   C. 98°-100° Fahrenheit.

   D. 97°-99° Fahrenheit.

59. If skin comes into contact with chemical or biological germs, the first thing to do is

   A. wait to wash skin until you leave the patient's room.

   B. wash the skin after you are done treating the patient.

   C. wipe skin with a cloth.

   D. wash skin immediately.

60. MRSA is a drug resistant

   A. virus.

   B. fungus.

   C. nonpathogen.

   D. bacteria.

ANSWER KEY AND EXPLANATIONS

1. B	11. D	21. B	31. D	41. A	51. A
2. D	12. B	22. A	32. C	42. B	52. A
3. D	13. D	23. C	33. D	43. C	53. C
4. D	14. D	24. C	34. C	44. B	54. B
5. C	15. C	25. A	35. B	45. B	55. D
6. A	16. C	26. C	36. A	46. C	56. A
7. A	17. A	27. A	37. D	47. B	57. C
8. C	18. B	28. C	38. B	48. A	58. D
9. A	19. A	29. A	39. B	49. B	59. D
10. D	20. C	30. C	40. A	50. D	60. D

1. **The correct answer is B.** The food pyramid is the guide that represents the standards of good nutrition in the United States. DASH dietary guidelines (choice A) are healthy heart eating plans created for those who have high blood pressure. The National Health and Nutrition Examination Survey (NHANES) (choice C) is a program designed to study and evaluate the health and nutritional level of the U.S. population. The United States Department of Agriculture (USDA) is the agency that regulates meat, poultry, and egg products.

2. **The correct answer is D.** The right way to perform the Heimlich maneuver on a choking person is to, first, make a fist, then place the thumb side against the abdomen, and rapidly thrust upward. Pushing down while laying the hands flat on the abdomen (choice A), quickly pushing downward while pressing one fist against the abdomen (choice B), and tenderly thrusting downward with the fist (choice C) are all incorrect ways to perform the Heimlich maneuver.

3. **The correct answer is D.** Hyperextension is the excessive straightening of a body part. Flexion (choice A) decreases the angle when bending a body part, while extension (choice B) increases the angle between two body parts. Dorsiflexion (choice C) is the backward bending of the wrist or foot.

4. **The correct answer is D.** Since cranks are used to lower and raise the head and foot of the bed and to control the height of the bed, it is important to fold the cranks under the bed when all the adjustments have been made. Turning the cranks clockwise to lock the bed (choice A) and turning the cranks counterclockwise to unlock the bed (choice B) are not the proper functions of the cranks. It is not the best option to always have the patient's head elevated (choice C).

5. **The correct answer is C.** A pen and paper or a typing device are the best tools to use for someone who is completely deaf. The aide projecting their voice as loud as possible (choice A) or using a system of alarm rings (choice B) are best options for those who have some hearing abilities. The Braille notation system (choice D) is used for those who are blind.

6. **The correct answer is A.** A physician is asking for a complete blood count if they are looking for the CBC. There is no such thing as a complete blood catheter (choice B) nor a center for blood diseases (choice C). The center for blood disorders (choice D) is a facility that cares for those with blood disorders.

7. **The correct answer is A.** Dressings should always be clean and dry because bacteria can multiply in moisture and cause significant infection. To limit the exposure to bacteria, the patient's dressing

should not air dry (choice B). A dressing does not always have to be fastened by tape (choice C) nor should the dressing be close-fitting to keep out bacteria (choice D).

8. **The correct answer is C.** Disinfection is the process of killing all harmful viruses and bacteria on all surfaces. Sanitation (choice A) relates to cleaning up waste. The clean technique (choice B) does not get rid of viruses and bacteria but reduces the transmission of them. Handwashing (choice D) is a way to get rid of viruses or bacteria on hands but not on all surfaces.

9. **The correct answer is A.** Cognitive impairment can range from mild to severe for a resident who has trouble recalling, learning new things, focusing, or making everyday life decisions. Developmental disorder (choice B) is a category of mental health conditions that mainly affect learning, recall, perception, and problem solving. Motor skill disorders (choice C) appear in children that seem to have extremely poor coordination. Alzheimer's disease (choice D) is a permanent developmental brain disorder that slowly destroys memory and thinking skills.

10. **The correct answer is D.** Policies and procedures are the written guidelines for the care of the residents and the operation of a healthcare facility. Grievances (choice A) are a formal complaint filed by a resident about their care or living space. Involuntary confinement (choice B) is physically preventing a resident from leaving a room or area. An informed consent (choice C) is the permission granted by a resident after understanding the risks, benefits, and alternatives to a procedure or treatment plan.

11. **The correct answer is D.** Vital signs measure basic functions like blood pressure, temperature, and pulse. A stethoscope (choice A), a thermometer (choice B), and an otoscope (choice C) are devices used to measure vital signs.

12. **The correct answer is B.** Flatus is gas in the intestinal tract or that which is passed through the anus. Fascia (choice A) is a flat band of tissue below the skin that covers underlying tissues

and separates different layers of tissue. Fantod (choice C) is a state of anxiety or an irritable outburst. Facies (choice D) is a distinctive facial expression or appearance linked with a specific medical condition.

13. **The correct answer is D.** Dementia is caused by different diseases that affect the brain. Alzheimer's disease (choice A), in which plaques and tangles develop inside the brain, is the most common cause of dementia. Depression (choice B) is a mood disorder caused by constant sadness. Bi-polar disorder (choice C) is a mental disorder that causes extreme mood shifts.

14. **The correct answer is D.** Sterilization of medical instruments is the process used in destroying all pathogens contained on them. Combustion (choice A) is the process of burning something. The clean technique (choice B) does not get rid of viruses and bacteria but reduces the transmission of them. Autoclaves (choice C) are steam sterilizers used to kill harmful bacteria.

15. **The correct answer is C.** The nursing assistant should politely listen to the patient who wants to share a religious experience but should move on when the opportunity presents itself. Sitting and listening for as long as it takes (choice A) can interfere with a nursing assistant's responsibilities to other patients, so knowing when to move on will be important. Stating that you are not allowed to discuss religion (choice B) and telling them you are busy with another patient (choice D) goes against the roles and responsibilities of the nursing assistant.

16. **The correct answer is C.** Since all blood spills are treated as possibly infectious, the first thing to do is clear out the area to avoid anyone else interacting with the broken glass or spill. Standard precautions apply here, so calling in the nurse to pick up the broken glass while the aide tends to the patient (choice A), calling 911 and housekeeping (choice B), and treating the patient at the site of accident (choice C) are not the protocols to follow.

17. **The correct answer is A.** Pronation is turning the arms and palms downward or foot inward. The act

of facing the arms or palms upward is supination (choice B). Rotation (choice C) is the turning or circling around something. Opposition (choice D) is moving the thumb, while crossing the palm, to the other fingers in the hand.

18. **The correct answer is B.** Standard precautions are necessary while delivering care to patients regardless of how sick they are. When a patient is known to have a very contagious illness, contact precautions (choice A) and/or transmission precautions (choice C) are used in addition to standard precautions. Airborne precautions (choice D) need to be used for illnesses that are spread by the air.

19. **The correct answer is A.** A urinary tract infection is commonly acquired when a person is in a healthcare facility. Shingles (choice B), human papilloma virus (choice C), and chicken pox (choice D) are not typically acquired in a healthcare facility.

20. **The correct answer is C.** Regression is a patient's defense mechanism used to relieve stress by returning to immature behavior. Rationalization (choice A) is a defense mechanism that uses an excuse to justify a behavior. Projection (choice B) is a defense mechanism that sees behaviors or feelings in others that are one's own. Repression (choice D) is a defense mechanism used to block painful thoughts or feelings from entering one's mind.

21. **The correct answer is B.** Any serious illness or injury needing a prompt response requires a call to emergency medical services. A patient whose injuries or illnesses do not require a prompt response can wait for 24 hours (choice A), visit the urgent care (choice C), or visit the primary care physician (choice D).

22. **The correct answer is A.** A local emergency system phone number is not on most warning labels because there is a commonly known national emergency phone number (911). Most warning labels list the health and physical hazards (choice B), the protective gear to wear (choice C), and the storage and disposal information (choice D).

23. **The correct answer is C.** Handwashing for a CNA should last for at least 20 seconds. Washing hands for 10 seconds (choice B) is not as effective in getting rid of germs. Although washing hands for at least 30 seconds (choice A) was once standard, it is now standard to wash hands for 20 seconds. Although 60 seconds (choice D) will get rid of the germs, it is not the basic recommended amount of time.

24. **The correct answer is C.** A patient who takes medication on an as-needed basis will have PRN written in the chart. A chart with QD (choice A), BID (choice B), and TID (choice D) written means that the patient is taking the medication once daily, twice daily, and three times daily, respectively.

25. **The correct answer is A.** A patient with Alzheimer's disease cannot cope well when they are unable to communicate their needs. An Alzheimer's patient may be disoriented (choice B), confused (choice C), and combative (choice D) because they are agitated and unable to communicate their needs.

26. **The correct answer is C.** A DNR order is written by a physician instructing all healthcare providers not to revive a patient if the heart stops or they stop breathing. Fall risk is noted in a patient's chart if they are at risk of falling (choice A). Brain death is when the brain has no function (choice B). Unless there is an advance directive or a DNR order, legally, a patient will need to be revived (choice D).

27. **The correct answer is A.** Respiratory rate measures the number of breaths taken per minute while the body is at rest. The metabolic rate (choice B) is the number of calories the body burns in a day while resting. Heart rate (choice C) measures how many times the heart beats per minute. Mortality rate (choice D) is the number of deaths in a specific population compared to the general population.

28. **The correct answer is C.** Since addiction changes the addict's brain chemistry, it allows them to lose control of their behaviors. The ideas that addiction

changes only the behavior of the addict (choice A), changes only the physical appearance of the addict (choice B) and changes no one (choice D) are false.

29. **The correct answer is A.** Individuals with anti-social personalities are charming and fun, but they also fail to take responsibility, violate other's rights, and lack remorse. Patients with borderline personality disorder (choice B) have a problem managing their emotions. Patients with histrionic personality disorder (choice C) have extreme attention-seeking and drama type emotions. Patients with schizotypal personality disorder (choice D) have unusual, magical-thinking behaviors.

30. **The correct answer is C.** After a needle stick, always wash the area off with soap and warm water for multiple minutes. Reporting it to the nurse (choice A) happens after washing the area. Never attempt to pinch the blood out (choice B) to avoid any possible contamination. Applying hand sanitizer and ointment (choice D) does not allow for any possible pathogens to be washed away from the skin.

31. **The correct answer is D.** Soap should be applied after wetting the hands. To help keep germs from spreading, soap should not be applied before wetting the hands (choice A), before setting the water temperature (choice B), or after taking off the gloves (choice C).

32. **The correct answer is C.** Paraplegia is the inability to move the bottom half of the body. Cardioplegia (choice A) is the paralysis of the heart. Hemiplegia (choice B) is paralysis on one side of the body. Quadriplegia (choice D) is the paralysis of all the extremities.

33. **The correct answer is D.** Listening is the most effective tool in resolving a resident's conflict because it allows the aide to understand the concern and address it. Poor communication (choice A), feeling misunderstood (choice B), and making assumptions (choice C) are ways conflicts can arise with a resident.

34. **The correct answer is C.** A provider should always look at the ID bracelet first to accurately identify a patient. Asking a family member (choice A) or waiting for a nurse (choice B) to identify a patient can be an option after looking at the patient's ID bracelet first. A provider should never treat a patient (choice D) before looking at an ID bracelet.

35. **The correct answer is B.** An incident report is used to record the details of an unusual situation that occurs in a facility. Risk management (choice A) identifies the potential problems in a situation. An audit report (choice C) is a formal opinion sharing the correctness or quality of information given by a facility. Prevention assessment (choice D) is a tool used to identify a problem before it happens.

36. **The correct answer is A.** Since the body needs to be washed first and the genital and rectal areas last, the basin needs to cleaned first and the water replaced. Replacing the washcloth (choice B) occurs after the basin is cleaned first and the water replaced. Helping the patient bathe allows her to see the proper bath technique without reminding her that a bath begins with the face (choice C). Since the water in the basin is contaminated, it is policy and procedure not to add a disinfectant to the dirty water and continue bathing (choice D).

37. **The correct answer is D.** CNAs should note that Americans view direct eye contact as a way of showing honesty and candidness. In Middle Eastern cultures, direct eye contact can be perceived as rudeness, hostility, or sexual aggressiveness (choice A). In some Asian and Native American cultures, direct eye contact can be perceived as disrespectful or rude (choices B and C).

38. **The correct answer is B.** *Cognition* is defined as the brain skills and the mental activities needed to carry out tasks. Intelligence is the ability to apply knowledge (choice A). Intelligence Quotient (IQ) tests are designed to assess your overall ability to solve problems and understand concepts (choice C). Cognitive psychology is the science of how we think, learn, focus, solve problems, forget, and remember (choice D).

39. **The correct answer is B.** A soft toothette is best used when a patient is unconscious to avoid

problems with aspirations of fluids or toothpaste. Having dentures (choice A), complaining of a toothache (choice C), and having a seizure (choice D) are not necessarily the best situations in which to use a toothette.

40. **The correct answer is A.** It is very important to fully dry the entire body in order to avoid moist areas where bacterial growth and skin breakdown can occur. Pat drying the body (choice B), applying lotion between the fingers and toes (choice C), and air drying (choice D) allows moisture to remain on the skin and creates a risk for bacterial growth and breakdown of the skin.

41. **The correct answer is A.** Keeping the patient's spine aligned while turning or moving them is log rolling. The dorsal recumbent position keeps the head and shoulders slightly elevated with a pillow (choice B). The Bozeman's position supports the knee-elbow position with straps (choice C). The Fowler's position keeps the head of the patient's bed raised 30-90 degrees above the level with the knees sometimes elevated (choice D).

42. **The correct answer is B.** The process of transferring becomes longer rather than shorter because the gait belt is there to aid the CNA. Without the assistance of the gait belt, there is an increased chance that the aide will strain their back (choice A), use more energy (choice C), and run the risk of a patient falling (choice D).

43. **The correct answer is C.** Rolling the eyes is a non-verbal form of communication that can send a negative message to a patient. A smile (choice A) and a gentle touch on the shoulder (choice B) are positive forms of non-verbal communication. A sarcastic response (choice D), although negative, is a verbal form of communication.

44. **The correct answer is B.** Since tears do not contain blood or pathogens in large amounts, they are not considered infectious. Plasma (choice A), vaginal discharge (choice C), and saliva (choice D) are highly infectious.

45. **The correct answer is B.** A person is incoherent when their conversation is chaotic without logical connection or direct relevance. A tranquil (choice

A) patient is calm when in conversation. A vague (choice C) patient lacks the ability to be focused in conversation. A flat (choice D) patient lacks emotional expression in conversation.

46. **The correct answer is C.** Although a CNA cannot dress the wound, it is within their scope of practice to assist in the process. Since a CNA can only assist a nurse in dressing the wound, receiving permission to dress the wound (choice A) is not an option. Having the patient move to a new position (choice B) can occur after the wound has been dressed. A CNA can document their own observations (choice D) and does not need the nurse to do that.

47. **The correct answer is B.** HIPAA are federal laws that allow healthcare providers to share appropriate patient information with those directly involved in caring for them. Healthcare providers who share patient health information without the expressed consent of the patient, whether with the family (choice A) or the spouse (choice B), are in violation of the HIPAA federal laws. Failure to share relevant medical information (choice D) with concerned parties is also a violation of HIPAA standards.

48. **The correct answer is A.** Since moving into a long-term facility can be a difficult transition, having the right to possess personal items in their room is helpful to the elderly person. Having the items the facility says they can possess (choice B) and choosing the items donated by the local thrift store (choice C) do not provide the elderly with reasonable options that will ease their transition. Requesting specific items of their choosing to be paid for by the long-term facility (choice D) is not part of the options offered by a long-term facility.

49. **The correct answer is B.** Tympanic temperature is measured by inserting a thermometer in the ear. Rectal temperature (choice A) is measured by inserting a thermometer in the rectum. Temporal temperature (choice C) is measured by using a scanner across the forehead. Axillary temperature (choice D) is measured by placing a thermometer under the armpit.

50. **The correct answer is D.** Nodding encouragingly as someone speaks is an example of positive body language. Having eyes wide open with a smile (choice A) can come across as patronizing. Shrugging shoulders up (choice B) can come across as confused or not interested. Staring at a person with a puzzled look (choice D) can demonstrate confusion and be discouraging.

51. **The correct answer is A.** Restraints use physical force to restrict a patient's freedom with or without consent. Rationale for restraints (choice B) is a set of reasons necessary for when a patient is in immediate danger or a danger to others. Documentation of restraints (choice C) are carefully written standards that meet the need to restrain someone. Restrain assessment (choice D) is the process of checking in on the patient's physical health while they are confined.

52. **The correct answer A.** To minimize choking, it is important to give quadriplegics small bites of food and permit enough time to chew the food. Giving fluids after the meal (choice B), rushing through the meal (choice C), and dressing and grooming the resident at the same time (choice D) does not allow a resident to wash down food and can pose a choking hazard.

53. **The correct answer is C.** It is important to check for a bleeding problem by asking the nurse and looking in the patient's record. Beginning at the sideburns and shaving sideways (choice A) and shaving downward on the neck (choice B) are incorrect ways to shave someone and can lead to cuts and nicks. Unless it is stated in a patient's record, it is not necessary to have someone assist you (choice D).

54. **The correct answer is B.** Making sure to carry the dirty linen away from the body helps to minimize contact with bodily fluids and is a proper way to handle the dirty linen. Wearing gloves only when changing linen (choice A), placing dirty linen next to clean linen (choice C), and disposing of dirty linen in the normal trash (choice D) are improper ways to handle dirty linen and help to spread infection.

55. **The correct answer is D.** For safety and liability reasons, doctors or nurses are the practitioners typically given the responsibility to cut toenails. For the same liability reasons, nursing assistants (choice A), family members (choice B), and physical therapists (choice C) are discouraged from cutting a resident's toenails.

56. **The correct answer is A.** A patient cannot have anything by mouth if NPO is written in the chart. If NKDA is written in the chart, then there is no known drug allergy (choice B). If no solid food (choice C) is written in the chart, then a liquid diet option is provided. If NKFA is written in the chart, then there is no known food allergy (choice D).

57. **The correct answer is C.** Disinfection kills just the pathogens. Sterilization destroys the nonpathogens (choice A) and the microbes (choice B), not disinfection. Sterilization destroys of all the microbes, as well as the pathogens and nonpathogens (choice D).

58. **The correct answer is D.** The normal temperature range is 97°-99° Fahrenheit. All the other ranges—95°-97° Fahrenheit (choice A), 100°-101° Fahrenheit (choice B), and 98°-100° Fahrenheit (choice C)—are incorrect.

59. **The correct answer is D.** Washing skin immediately after being exposed to chemical or biological germs is the first thing that should be done. Waiting to wash skin until you leave the patient's room (choice A), washing the skin after you are done treating the patient (choice B), and wiping the skin with a cloth (choice C) are ways to spread the chemical or biological germs.

60. **The correct answer is D.** MRSA is a drug-resistant bacterium found on a patient's skin. MRSA is not a virus (choice A), a fungus (choice B), or a nonpathogen (choice C).

NOTES

PRACTICE TEST

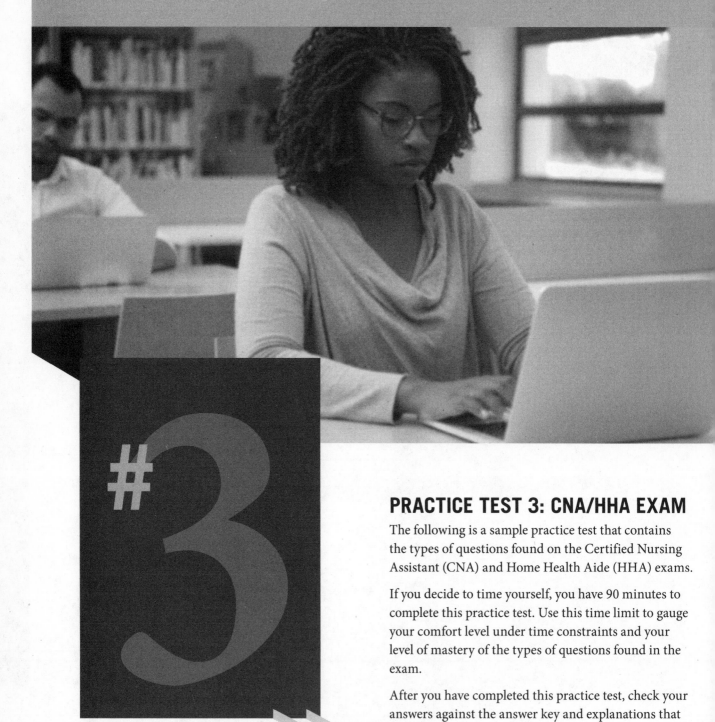

#3

PRACTICE TEST 3: CNA/HHA EXAM

The following is a sample practice test that contains the types of questions found on the Certified Nursing Assistant (CNA) and Home Health Aide (HHA) exams.

If you decide to time yourself, you have 90 minutes to complete this practice test. Use this time limit to gauge your comfort level under time constraints and your level of mastery of the types of questions found in the exam.

After you have completed this practice test, check your answers against the answer key and explanations that follow the test.

PRACTICE TEST 3: CNA/HHA EXAM ANSWER SHEET

1. Ⓐ Ⓑ Ⓒ Ⓓ
2. Ⓐ Ⓑ Ⓒ Ⓓ
3. Ⓐ Ⓑ Ⓒ Ⓓ
4. Ⓐ Ⓑ Ⓒ Ⓓ
5. Ⓐ Ⓑ Ⓒ Ⓓ
6. Ⓐ Ⓑ Ⓒ Ⓓ
7. Ⓐ Ⓑ Ⓒ Ⓓ
8. Ⓐ Ⓑ Ⓒ Ⓓ
9. Ⓐ Ⓑ Ⓒ Ⓓ
10. Ⓐ Ⓑ Ⓒ Ⓓ
11. Ⓐ Ⓑ Ⓒ Ⓓ
12. Ⓐ Ⓑ Ⓒ Ⓓ
13. Ⓐ Ⓑ Ⓒ Ⓓ
14. Ⓐ Ⓑ Ⓒ Ⓓ
15. Ⓐ Ⓑ Ⓒ Ⓓ

16. Ⓐ Ⓑ Ⓒ Ⓓ
17. Ⓐ Ⓑ Ⓒ Ⓓ
18. Ⓐ Ⓑ Ⓒ Ⓓ
19. Ⓐ Ⓑ Ⓒ Ⓓ
20. Ⓐ Ⓑ Ⓒ Ⓓ
21. Ⓐ Ⓑ Ⓒ Ⓓ
22. Ⓐ Ⓑ Ⓒ Ⓓ
23. Ⓐ Ⓑ Ⓒ Ⓓ
24. Ⓐ Ⓑ Ⓒ Ⓓ
25. Ⓐ Ⓑ Ⓒ Ⓓ
26. Ⓐ Ⓑ Ⓒ Ⓓ
27. Ⓐ Ⓑ Ⓒ Ⓓ
28. Ⓐ Ⓑ Ⓒ Ⓓ
29. Ⓐ Ⓑ Ⓒ Ⓓ
30. Ⓐ Ⓑ Ⓒ Ⓓ

31. Ⓐ Ⓑ Ⓒ Ⓓ
32. Ⓐ Ⓑ Ⓒ Ⓓ
33. Ⓐ Ⓑ Ⓒ Ⓓ
34. Ⓐ Ⓑ Ⓒ Ⓓ
35. Ⓐ Ⓑ Ⓒ Ⓓ
36. Ⓐ Ⓑ Ⓒ Ⓓ
37. Ⓐ Ⓑ Ⓒ Ⓓ
38. Ⓐ Ⓑ Ⓒ Ⓓ
39. Ⓐ Ⓑ Ⓒ Ⓓ
40. Ⓐ Ⓑ Ⓒ Ⓓ
41. Ⓐ Ⓑ Ⓒ Ⓓ
42. Ⓐ Ⓑ Ⓒ Ⓓ
43. Ⓐ Ⓑ Ⓒ Ⓓ
44. Ⓐ Ⓑ Ⓒ Ⓓ
45. Ⓐ Ⓑ Ⓒ Ⓓ

46. Ⓐ Ⓑ Ⓒ Ⓓ
47. Ⓐ Ⓑ Ⓒ Ⓓ
48. Ⓐ Ⓑ Ⓒ Ⓓ
49. Ⓐ Ⓑ Ⓒ Ⓓ
50. Ⓐ Ⓑ Ⓒ Ⓓ
51. Ⓐ Ⓑ Ⓒ Ⓓ
52. Ⓐ Ⓑ Ⓒ Ⓓ
53. Ⓐ Ⓑ Ⓒ Ⓓ
54. Ⓐ Ⓑ Ⓒ Ⓓ
55. Ⓐ Ⓑ Ⓒ Ⓓ
56. Ⓐ Ⓑ Ⓒ Ⓓ
57. Ⓐ Ⓑ Ⓒ Ⓓ
58. Ⓐ Ⓑ Ⓒ Ⓓ
59. Ⓐ Ⓑ Ⓒ Ⓓ
60. Ⓐ Ⓑ Ⓒ Ⓓ

PRACTICE TEST 3: CNA/HHA EXAM

90 minutes—60 questions

Directions: Read each question below and choose the correct answer from the four choices provided. Only one choice is correct, so choose carefully.

---

1. In culturally understanding how patients deal with pain, it is best to NOT

   A. explore religious attitudes that impact the meaning of pain.

   B. recognize how cultures react and display pain in varied ways.

   C. use the traditional 0-10 pain scale.

   D. be familiar with how cultures find relief from pain.

2. An act NOT part of the daily roles and responsibility of a nurse's aide is to

   A. provide privacy and encourage independence as much as possible.

   B. share deeply personal and financial information with the resident.

   C. check the resident's care plan.

   D. observe the resident for pain, discomfort, and fatigue.

3. Bending knees, keeping a straight back, and tightening stomach muscles are safe ways to do a(n)

   A. balancing technique.

   B. awkward posture.

   C. proper lifting technique.

   D. massage technique.

4. In an infection, a reservoir is

   A. where the germ lives and grows.

   B. a body opening that allows the germ to penetrate.

   C. a body opening that allows the germ to exit.

   D. a germ.

5. A patient who is extremely suspicious or believes they are being persecuted is suffering from

   A. grandiosity.

   B. logic.

   C. paranoia.

   D. euphoria.

6. An advance directive is

   A. the rule that healthcare providers can only share appropriate patient information with those directly involved in caring for them.

   B. the idea that an individual's personal information is protected from public examination.

   C. a do not resuscitate order.

   D. a legal document indicating end-of-life decisions ahead of time.

7. What is an activity of daily living that a CNA does NOT perform?

   A. Bathing

   B. Dressing

   C. Toileting

   D. Cooking

8. Slowing down disease and disability, keeping cognitive and physical behaviors, and continuing to be actively connected with life is the best possible way for

   A. primary aging.

   B. secondary aging.

   C. successful aging.

   D. geriatrics.

9. Reliable and consistent steps taken prior to performing any activity with a patient are

   A. secondary.

   B. tertiary.

   C. initial.

   D. final.

10. To help lessen pressure sores on bony prominences for a bed-ridden patient, it is best to

    A. use a special bed.

    B. reposition the patient at the start of every shift.

    C. prop the area by using a few pillows.

    D. use extra blankets.

11. A communication professional who mediates between different speakers of language is a(n)

    A. linguist.

    B. interpreter.

    C. polyglot.

    D. signer.

12. When nurse aides interact with patients, they should remember that

    A. a big portion of communication is nonverbal.

    B. patients lose their ability to communicate as they get older.

    C. oral communication is the most effective way of communicating.

    D. communication boards are ineffective ways to convey something.

13. While helping a confused resident to dress, the resident consistently reaches for the comb several times. The aide should

    A. gently grab the comb and place it in a drawer.

    B. place the comb in a back pocket.

    C. let the resident hold the comb.

    D. finish dressing the resident quickly.

14. Which is NOT a body position?

    A. Supine

    B. Prone

    C. Lateral

    D. Contract

15. Which is an example of a simple carbohydrate?

    A. Nuts

    B. Black beans

    C. Baked potato

    D. Steel oats

16. A stethoscope is a piece of medical equipment used to

    A. look at the inside of the ear.

    B. look at the mouth and throat.

    C. listen to sounds made by the inside of the body.

    D. test the knee jerk reflex.

17. A fast heart rate in an adult that is greater than 100 beats per minute (bpm) is called

    A. tachycardia.

    B. bradycardia.

    C. arrhythmia.

    D. atrial fibrillation.

18. During a patient's bath, the nurse's aide realizes there are not enough bath towels to dry the patient. The aide should

    A. ask the patient to utilize a towel previously used.

    B. ask the patient to hold on while they run to get a towel.

    C. ask a co-worker to bring a fresh towel.

    D. use a fresh hand towel that is next to them.

19. All of these are common handwashing procedures EXCEPT:

   A. Drying hands with paper towels

   B. Using friction and getting between fingers

   C. Lathering with soap for 20 or more seconds

   D. Rinsing them in hot water

20. When a resident is not accepting loss well, the best way an aide can help is to

   A. allow the resident to grieve privately.

   B. encourage the resident to accept the loss.

   C. take them off the attendance list of social activities and meeting groups.

   D. encourage the resident to discuss the loss.

21. While moving, the safe way to use the body to maintain balance, posture, and alignment is called

   A. ergonomics.

   B. body mechanics.

   C. anthropometric measurements.

   D. ambulation.

22. An ombudsman is a(n)

   A. person who dispenses medications and gives treatment.

   B. official who is appointed as an advocate or go-between for a patient.

   C. person who provides activities of daily living for a patient.

   D. person who manages, coordinates, and delivers skilled nursing care.

23. After spending the day with family, the resident returns with bruises. The CNA notices and is required to

   A. mention it right away to the family.

   B. share it with the resident's roommate.

   C. report the bruising to the licensed nurse.

   D. monitor more closely for any changes.

24. Influenza is a highly contagious _____ infection.

   A. parasitic

   B. viral

   C. bacterial

   D. fungal

25. If a patient has an airborne infection and is transported to occupational therapy, they should wear

   A. shields.

   B. gloves.

   C. a mask.

   D. a gown.

26. If a nursing assistant notices a patient is struggling to have spiritual needs met, a form of care that should be offered is ensuring that

   A. medical care is prioritized.

   B. the patient cannot express their feelings.

   C. there is not a way for religious rituals to be practiced.

   D. there is contact between the patient and a religious or spiritual advisor.

27. The proper order of putting on personal protective equipment (PPE) is

   A. mask, gown, goggles, gloves.

   B. goggles, mask, gloves, gown.

   C. gloves, goggles, gown, mask.

   D. gown, mask, goggles, gloves.

28. Unable to get an interpreter but needing to communicate with a resident who speaks another language, a CNA should

   A. come back when the interpreter is available.

   B. listen to the resident and say nothing.

   C. use gestures and/or communication boards.

   D. speak calmly and deliberately with the hopes that the resident will understand.

29. A bed-bound patient should be repositioned every

    A. 5 hours.

    B. 4 hours.

    C. 6 hours.

    D. 2 hours.

30. When an evacuation is required, the people rescued first are those who are

    A. nearest to the outside door.

    B. able to walk.

    C. closest to the fire.

    D. panicking.

31. Physical therapy

    A. is a person who is a movement expert and improves the quality of life of their patients through exercise.

    B. is the care received to help ease pain and provide better fine motor and cognitive skills.

    C. is the care received to help ease pain and provide better gross motor function.

    D. assists with depression and other mental disorders.

32. The aging condition where the joint cartilage breaks down over time causing pain, stiffness, and swelling is

    A. osteoarthritis.

    B. rheumatoid arthritis.

    C. osteoporosis.

    D. Paget's disease.

33. The Heimlich maneuver is used when a person is

    A. dehydrated.

    B. choking.

    C. having an anaphylactic allergy attack.

    D. having a panic attack.

34. An addictive chemical found in tobacco is

    A. adrenaline.

    B. nicotine.

    C. cannabis.

    D. opioid.

35. Each state certification board presents a list of activities that describes the CNA's

    A. scope of practice.

    B. salary.

    C. experience.

    D. benefits.

36. When preparing a patient's room, a nursing assistant should perform all of these EXCEPT:

    A. Dispense the necessary medications

    B. Adjust the lighting

    C. Check for easy accessibility to the call bell

    D. Adjust the back rest

37. Lewy body dementia is known for

    A. being the most common form of dementia.

    B. occurring after a stroke.

    C. causing visual hallucinations during the early stages.

    D. causing changes in appetite during the early stages.

38. A law passed by the government to institute basic standards of care and rights for those living in nursing homes is

    A. the healthcare proxy.

    B. the Occupational Safety and Health Administration (OSHA).

    C. the Omnibus Budget Reconciliation Act (OBRA).

    D. Medicare.

39. Morning care refers to care

    A. given after breakfast.

    B. offered while eating breakfast.

    C. offered after noon.

    D. given before breakfast.

40. A chemical or diseased waste that is harmful to humans must be disposed in a container labeled

   A. waste.

   B. caution.

   C. hazard.

   D. biohazard.

41. The type of exercise that allows an increased range of joint movement is

   A. aerobic.

   B. strength.

   C. endurance.

   D. stretching.

42. Patients who are carriers are

   A. people who transmit disease but are asymptomatic.

   B. people who transmit disease and are symptomatic.

   C. people who are sick but do not transmit disease.

   D. any organism that lives on dead organic matter.

43. The physical contact between an infected patient and a susceptible patient is

   A. indirect contact.

   B. direct contact.

   C. indirect contact exposure.

   D. direct contact exposure.

44. An extremely low body temperature where the body loses heat faster than it can make it is

   A. hyperthermia.

   B. heat stroke.

   C. hypothermia.

   D. hypothyroidism.

45. The hospital's primary accrediting body is the

   A. Joint Commission on Accreditation of Health-care Organizations (JCAHO).

   B. National Committee for Quality Assurance (NCQA).

   C. Occupational Safety and Health Administration (OSHA).

   D. Commission on Dental Accreditation (CDA).

46. When an aide provides peri-care to a female patient, it is important to wash from front to back to avoid spreading bacteria from the patient's

   A. vulva.

   B. vaginal sphincter.

   C. rectum.

   D. urethral meatus.

47. Since a resident wants to dine independently but is living with Parkinson's disease, the aide allows them to

   A. eat with lightweight utensils.

   B. eat with adaptive cutlery.

   C. eat with fingers.

   D. be fed by a volunteer.

48. The aide's response to a charge nurse who asks them to remove a patient's catheter should be to

   A. remove the catheter.

   B. ask for instructions on how to remove a catheter.

   C. remind the nurse that it is not within the aide's scope of practice.

   D. request that another aide assist them with the removal of the catheter.

49. Phobias are a type of

   A. mood disorder.

   B. anxiety disorder.

   C. aversion therapy.

   D. panic attack.

50. "What can I change to get the outcome I want?" is a question commonly asked during which stage of the grieving process?

   A. Denial

   B. Anger

   C. Bargaining

   D. Acceptance

51. A Doppler device is used to detect a

   A. fever.

   B. heartbeat.

   C. metabolic rate.

   D. respiration rate.

52. If a home health assistant is endangered or uncomfortable in a home setting, they should

   A. try to resolve the situation by staying at the home.

   B. confront the person who is causing the problem.

   C. inform the nurse about the matter.

   D. continue to provide care and disregard the situation.

53. An elderly patient's constant exposure to urine and feces commonly causes

   A. skin irritation and breakdown.

   B. waterlogging.

   C. incontinence.

   D. dry skin.

54. The inability to understand spoken or written words is

   A. anomic aphagia.

   B. dysphagia.

   C. receptive aphagia.

   D. expressive aphagia.

55. The body's ability to resist infection is its

   A. antibodies.

   B. immunity.

   C. nonpathogen.

   D. pH balance.

56. Gear worn to reduce the exposure of germs that can cause serious workplace illness or injury is

   A. personal protective equipment.

   B. biohazard signs.

   C. medical equipment.

   D. ambulatory equipment.

57. A tube used to drain urine from the bladder of all patients is a(n)

   A. enema.

   B. suppository.

   C. catheter.

   D. condom catheter.

58. The best way to minimize exposure to airborne germs for healthcare workers is to

   A. wear a gown.

   B. wear a mask.

   C. wash hands.

   D. wear a face shield.

59. To kill microbes in or on the body, the patient will have to take

   A. an antiseptic.

   B. antibiotics.

   C. minerals.

   D. an asepsis.

60. A patient who is trying to use verbal communication is using _____ to share information with others.

   A. cues

   B. sounds

   C. pictures

   D. facial and body movements

ANSWER KEY AND EXPLANATIONS

1. C	11. B	21. B	31. C	41. D	51. B
2. B	12. A	22. B	32. A	42. A	52. C
3. C	13. C	23. C	33. B	43. B	53. A
4. A	14. D	24. B	34. B	44. C	54. C
5. C	15. C	25. C	35. A	45. A	55. B
6. D	16. C	26. D	36. A	46. C	56. A
7. D	17. A	27. D	37. C	47. B	57. C
8. C	18. C	28. C	38. C	48. C	58. B
9. C	19. D	29. D	39. D	49. B	59. B
10. A	20. D	30. C	40. D	50. C	60. B

1. **The correct answer is C.** Since different cultures view pain in various ways, it is best not to use the traditional 0-10 pain scale but rather an alternative. In culturally understanding how patients deal with pain, exploring religious attitudes that impact the meaning of pain (choice A), recognizing how cultures react and display pain in varied ways (choice B), and being familiar with how cultures find relief from pain (choice D) would be insightful.

2. **The correct answer is B.** Sharing deeply personal and financial information with the resident is not an act that is part of the daily roles and responsibility of a nurse's aide. Providing privacy and encouraging independence as much as possible (choice A), checking the resident's care plan (choice C), and observing the resident for pain, discomfort, and fatigue (choice D) are all acts within the daily roles and responsibilities of a nurse's aide.

3. **The correct answer is C.** To limit strain and stress on the body while performing a proper lifting technique, it is important to bend the knees while keeping a straight back and tightening stomach muscles. Evenly distributing weight while holding the center of gravity is a balancing technique (choice A). Assuming an arrangement that places stress on the body is an awkward position (choice

B). The ability to use stretching and pressure in a regular pattern is a massage technique (choice D).

4. **The correct answer is A.** A reservoir is where the germ lives and multiplies. A body opening that allows the germ to penetrate (choice B) is a portal of entry. A body opening that allows the germ to leave (choice C) is a portal of exit. A germ (choice D) is also known as a pathogen.

5. **The correct answer is C.** Patients who suffer from paranoia are extremely suspicious of others and believe they are being persecuted. Patients who experience grandiosity (choice A) have an unrealistic sense of superiority. Logical (choice B) patients have sound and clear reasoning. Patients who are experiencing euphoria (choice D) have an intense happiness and feeling of greatness.

6. **The correct answer is D.** An advance directive legally allows a person to state their decisions about end-of-life care ahead of time. The Health Insurance Portability and Accountability Act (HIPAA) are federal laws which state that providers can only share appropriate patient information with those directly involved in caring for them (choice A). Privacy rights (choice B) ensure that an individual's personal information is protected from public examination. A do not resuscitate order (choice C) is written by a physician instructing all healthcare providers not to revive a patient if the heart stops or they stop breathing.

7. **The correct answer is D.** An instrumental activity of daily living not performed by a CNA is cooking. Bathing (choice A), dressing (choice B), and toileting (choice C) are all basic activities of daily living that CNAs provide assistance with.

8. **The correct answer is C.** Avoiding disease and disability, being actively connected to life, and maintaining healthy cognitive and physical behaviors is successful aging. Primary aging (choice A) includes the usual gradual changes in body systems that are experienced by everyone and not related to illness or disability. Secondary aging (choice B) includes unusual changes in body systems felt by some individuals but not all and related to disease or disability. Geriatrics (choice D) is the healthcare of the elderly.

9. **The correct answer is C.** For safety reasons, initial steps for any activity are to be taken before performing an activity with a patient. Secondary (choice A), tertiary (choice B), and final (choice D) steps are taken *after* making sure the reliable and consistent steps are initially performed for any activity.

10. **The correct answer is A.** The use of special beds that have high-density foam can help to lessen pressure sores on bony prominences. A patient should not be repositioned at the start of every shift (choice B) but every two hours. Although propping the patient by using a few pillows (choice C) and extra blankets (choice D) can be helpful, they are not the best options to avoid pressure sores.

11. **The correct answer is B.** An interpreter is a communication professional who mediates between speakers of different languages. A linguist (choice A) is a person who has studied languages. A polyglot (choice C) is a person who speaks, writes, and reads several languages. A signer (choice D) is a person who communicates by sign language.

12. **The correct answer is A.** Studies show that over 50% of all communication is nonverbal. Although some patients lose their ability to communicate as they get older (choice B), not all do. Oral communication is not always the most effective way of communicating (choice C). Communication

boards can be effective ways to convey something (choice D).

13. **The correct answer is C.** To be able to finish with the activity and minimize stress on the resident, a confused resident should be allowed to hold the comb. Gently grabbing the comb and placing it in a drawer (choice A), placing the comb in a back pocket (choice B), and quickly finishing with the resident's dressing (choice D) can seem rude and impersonal to a confused person.

14. **The correct answer is D.** "Contract" describes a muscle that becomes shorter and tighter, not a position of the body. The supine (choice A) position is when a patient is lying on their back. The prone (choice B) position is when a patient is lying on their stomach. The lateral (choice C) position is when a patient is lying on their side, left or right.

15. **The correct answer is C.** Potatoes are broken down by the body as a simple carbohydrate. Nuts (choice A), black beans (choice B), and steel oats (choice D) are all complex carbohydrates.

16. **The correct answer is C.** A stethoscope listens to the sounds made by the inside of the body. An otoscope looks at the inside of the ear (choice A). A tongue depressor looks at the mouth and throat (choice B). The hammer device is used to test the knee jerk reflex (choice D).

17. **The correct answer is A.** Tachycardia is a rapid heart rate greater than 100 bpm. Bradycardia (choice B) is a heart rate with less than 60 bpm. Arrhythmia (choice C) and atrial fibrillation (choice D) are abnormal erratic heart rates and rhythms.

18. **The correct answer is C.** Since a patient should never be left alone, asking a co-worker to get a towel is necessary. Asking the patient to utilize a towel previously used (choice A) is unsanitary. Asking the patient to hold on while the aide runs to get a towel (choice B) is unsafe. Using a fresh hand towel that is next to them (choice D) is not adequate to dry the body.

19. **The correct answer is D.** It is recommended to rinse hands in lukewarm water, not hot water. Drying hands with paper towels (choice A), using

friction and getting between fingers (choice B), and lathering with soap for 20 or more seconds (choice C) are all part of proper handwashing protocols.

20. **The correct answer is D.** Since each individual recovers from loss at a different pace, encouraging the resident to discuss their loss will allow them to move through the grieving process. Allowing the resident to grieve privately (choice A), encouraging the resident to accept the loss (choice B), and taking them off the attendance list of social activities and meeting groups (choice C) only promotes alienation and does not help them through the grieving process.

21. **The correct answer is B.** Body mechanics is the safe and proper use of the body. Ergonomics (choice A) is the study of people and their relationship with their work environment. Anthropometric measurements (choice C) are used to measure the form of the human body using BMI, height, and weight. Ambulation (choice D) is to walk about or move freely.

22. **The correct answer is B.** A person who acts as an advocate or a go-between for a patient is an ombudsman. A licensed practical nurse is a person who dispenses medications and gives treatment (choice A). A person who provides activities of daily living for a patient (choice C) is a nursing assistant. A registered nurse is a person who manages, coordinates, and delivers skilled nursing care (choice D).

23. **The correct answer is C.** The CNA is required to report any bruising to the licensed nurse. Mentioning it right away to the family (choice A), sharing it with the resident's roommate (choice B), and monitoring it closely for any changes (choice D) are all against the policies and procedures established at a facility.

24. **The correct answer is B.** Influenza, commonly known as the flu, is a viral infection that attacks the respiratory system. Influenza is not a parasitic (choice A), bacterial (choice C), or fungal (choice D) infection.

25. **The correct answer is C.** A mask, which protects the mouth and nose, should be worn by patients who have an airborne infection. Shields (choice A) prevent splatters from being transmitted. Gloves (choice B) prevent the hands from coming into physical contact with germs. Gowns (choice D) prevent the skin and clothing from coming into contact with germs.

26. **The correct answer is D.** Ensuring that there is contact between the patient and a religious or spiritual advisor is a way to help a patient have their spiritual needs met. Ensuring that medical care is more important (choice A), the patient cannot express their feelings (choice B), and there is not a way for religious rituals to be practiced (choice C) are not ways to meet the needs of a patient who is struggling spiritually.

27. **The correct answer is D.** Since PPE is an important part of infection control, the order—gown, mask, goggles, gloves—of putting it on is equally as important. The orders presented in choices A, B, and C could lead to infection exposure.

28. **The correct answer is C.** Using gestures and/or communication boards are simple ways to adjust and meet the immediate needs of the resident. Coming back when the interpreter is available (choice A) and listening to the resident and saying nothing (choice B) do not meet the immediate needs of the resident nor does it safeguard their client rights. Speaking calmly and deliberately with the hopes the resident understands you (choice D) can come across as demeaning, and it does not protect their client rights.

29. **The correct answer is D.** Repositioning a patient every 2 hours is the current recommended guidelines for care. Although repositioning can occur at 5 hours (choice A), 4 hours (choice B), and 6 hours (choice C), the current recommended guidelines state that a bed-bound patient should be repositioned every 2 hours.

30. **The correct answer is C.** Those closest to the fire are evacuated first. Depending on level of ability, those who are nearest to the outside door (choice A), those who can walk (choice B), and those who

are panicking will be rescued after those who are closest to the fire.

31. **The correct answer is C.** Physical therapy uses special exercises to help patients improve their physical abilities. A person who is a movement specialist and improves the quality of life of their patients through exercise (choice A) is a physical therapist. Occupational therapy is the care received to help ease pain and provide better fine motor and cognitive skills (choice B). Cognitive behavior therapy assists with depression and other mental disorders (choice D).

32. **The correct answer is A.** Osteoarthritis causes the joint cartilage to break down during the aging process. Rheumatoid arthritis (choice B) is where the immune system attacks joint tissue, causing inflammation, pain, swelling, and stiffness. Osteoporosis (choice C) is a loss of bone tissue usually due to hormonal changes. Paget's disease (choice D) is where there is an excessive amount of bone removal followed by additional larger bone formation that can result in pain and fracture.

33. **The correct answer is B.** When someone is choking, the Heimlich maneuver is applied. Intravenous fluids can be administered when someone is dehydrated (choice A). An EpiPen can be administered if someone is having an anaphylactic allergy attack (choice C). Anti-anxiety medication can be administered if someone is having a panic attack (choice D).

34. **The correct answer is B.** Nicotine is an addictive chemical found in the tobacco plant. Adrenaline (choice A) is a hormone released by the adrenal gland. Cannabis (choice C), which can create a dependence, comes from the hemp plant. Opioids (choice D), although addictive, are drugs used to treat severe pain.

35. **The correct answer is A.** The scope of practice for each state lists the duties a CNA can legally perform. Salary (choice B), experience (choice C), and benefits (choice D) are duties outside of the state board and belong with the facilities or organizations who hire CNA personnel.

36. **The correct answer is A.** CNAs are not allowed to dispense any medications; they must be administered by the nurse. Adjusting the lighting (choice B), checking for easy accessibility to the call bell (choice C), and adjusting the back rest (choice D) are all within the scope of duties of a CNA.

37. **The correct answer is C.** Visual hallucinations are one of the earliest signs of Lewy body dementia. Alzheimer's disease is the most common form of dementia (choice A). Vasculature dementia can develop after a stroke (choice B). One of the earliest forms of Parkinson's dementia is changes in appetite (choice D).

38. **The correct answer is C.** The Omnibus Budget Reconciliation Act (OBRA) provides basic standards of care and rights for those living in a nursing home. A healthcare proxy (choice A) is a document that gives someone, who is trusted, the ability to communicate healthcare decisions on behalf of someone that is unable to speak for themselves. Occupational Safety and Health Administration (OSHA) (choice B) is a government agency that makes rules to safeguard workers from dangers on the job. Medicare (choice D) is a federal health insurance program that primarily serves people who are over 65 years or younger people who are disabled.

39. **The correct answer is D.** Morning care refers to care given before breakfast. Morning care is typically not given after breakfast (choice A). Morning care is not offered to residents while they are eating breakfast (choice B) or after noon (choice C).

40. **The correct answer is D.** Biohazard waste has contaminated items and must be disposed of in a safe container labeled "biohazard." A waste (choice A) container is used for normal trash. A caution (choice B) or hazard (choice C) container is be used to demonstrate that there may be sensitive or dangerous items within them.

41. **The correct answer is D.** Stretching exercises allow an increased range of joint movement. Aerobic (choice A) exercise conditions the heart. Strength (choice B) exercises increase muscle strength. Endurance (choice D) exercises are any

level of physical activity that gives the body the ability to endure stress and hardship.

42. **The correct answer is A.** Carriers are people who transmit disease but do not show any symptoms. People who transmit disease and are symptomatic (choice B) are contagious. People who are sick but do not transmit disease (choice C) are symptomatic. Any organism that lives on dead organic matter (choice D) is a saprophyte.

43. **The correct answer is B.** A direct contact transmission occurs when a disease infected patient spreads a germ to a susceptible patient. Indirect contact (choice A) transmission occurs when germs can be spread through air and other means without direct human to human contact. Indirect contact exposure (choice C) occurs when a patient is visible to transmission from a reservoir or a vector. Direct contact exposure (choice D) is when a healthy patient is openly subjected to a patient who is infected.

44. **The correct answer is C.** Hypothermia is extremely low body temperature and is an emergency that can lead to death. Hyperthermia (choice A) is when the body experiences extremely high temperatures. Heat stroke (choice B), a form of hyperthermia, is when the body's core temperature is above 104° Fahrenheit. Hypothyroidism (choice D) is when the body does not create and distribute the thyroid hormone into the bloodstream possibly causing lower body temperatures.

45. **The correct answer is A.** The Joint Commission on Accreditation of Healthcare Organizations (JCAHO) accredits and certifies healthcare organizations, such as hospitals. The National Committee for Quality Assurance (NCQA) (choice B) accredits and certifies healthcare organizations comprised of providers, practices, and health plans. Occupational Safety and Health Administration (OSHA) (choice C) is a government agency that makes rules to safeguard workers from dangers on the job. The Commission on Dental Accreditation (CDA) (choice D) promotes the quality and improvement of dental education programs using standards.

46. **The correct answer is C.** Since the rectum is the source of fecal matter, wiping from front to back will avoid spreading bacteria. The vulva (choice A), vaginal sphincter (choice B), and urethral meatus (choice D) are all part of the vaginal structure and do not naturally come into contact with the fecal bacteria.

47. **The correct answer is B.** Adaptive cutlery is weighted, so it minimizes shaking in Parkinson's patients and allows them to eat more independently. Eating with lightweight utensils (choice A) will not help with the tremors from Parkinson's disease. Eating with fingers (choice C) is not sanitary. Being fed by a volunteer (choice D) does not allow for the level of independence the resident is requesting.

48. **The correct answer is C.** It is professionally appropriate to remind the nurse that it is not within an aide's scope of practice to remove a catheter. Therefore, removing the catheter (choice A), asking for instructions on how to remove a catheter (choice B), and requesting that another aide assist with the catheter removal (choice D) are tasks beyond the scope of practice of a CNA.

49. **The correct answer is B.** Phobias are a kind of anxiety disorder that cause irrational fear. Mood disorders (choice A) involve different ranges of feelings that can change the way a person feels or acts. Aversion therapy (choice C) is a treatment used to help a patient give up an unwanted behavior. Phobias can lead to a panic attack (choice D).

50. **The correct answer is C.** Grieving patients often ask this question during the bargaining stage of the grieving process. The denial stage (choice A) occurs beforehand usually and is rooted in the lack of acceptance of the situation. Both the anger stage (choice B) and the acceptance stage (choice D) come before and after bargaining, respectively. The anger stage is more emotional in nature, and the acceptance stage comes when the griever feels the most "at peace" since the grieving process started.

51. **The correct answer is B.** A Doppler device is a hand-held monitor that detects blood flow, pressure, and heartbeats. A fever (choice A) is detected by a thermometer. Calorimetry is used to measure metabolic rates (choice C). Respiratory rate (choice D) is measured by counting the number of breaths taken per minute while the body is at rest.

52. **The correct answer is C.** Informing the nurse is the first step to dealing with an uncomfortable or dangerous work situation for a home health assistant. Resolving the situation by staying at the home (choice A), confronting the person who is causing the problem (choice B), and disregarding the situation while continuing to provide care (choice D) are not the best solutions for maintaining a safe work environment.

53. **The correct answer is A.** If a patient has constant exposure to urine and feces, then skin irritation and breakdown is a common result. Feeling waterlogged (choice B) is when a patient has the feeling of an extraordinary amount of fluid in the abdomen, usually caused by bloating. Incontinence (choice C) is caused by the loss of bladder control. Dry skin (choice D) is a common result of aging.

54. **The correct answer is C.** Receptive aphagia is a language disorder which makes it hard for a person to understand spoken or written language. Anomic aphasia (choice A) is to have trouble using the right word for things, places, or events. Dysphagia (choice B) is difficulty with swallowing. Expressive aphagia (choice D) is the inability to speak or write out your thoughts clearly.

55. **The correct answer is B.** Immunity is the body's ability to resist infection. Antibodies (choice A) are proteins produced by the body's immune system when it receives harmful antigens. Nonpathogens

(choice C) are organisms that do not cause disease. The body's pH balance (choice D) is the level of acids and bases in the blood which help the body to function best.

56. **The correct answer is A.** Personal protective equipment is special gear used to protect workers from exposure to germs in a healthcare setting. Biohazard signs (choice B) are labels that indicate that there are contaminated items in a container.

57. **The correct answer is C.** A catheter is a tube used to drain urine from the bladder for all patients. An enema (choice A) is a liquid or gas that is inserted into the rectum to flush out the colon. A suppository (choice B) is a tube or cone typically placed in the rectum that releases medication and helps a bowel movement happen. A condom catheter (choice D) is a catheter that covers the penis and drains urine from the bladder.

58. **The correct answer is B.** Healthcare workers should always wear a mask to minimize contact with airborne germs. Wearing a gown (choice A), washing hands (choice C), and wearing a face shield (choice D) are not the best ways to protect healthcare workers from airborne germs.

59. **The correct answer is B.** Antibiotics fight to kill microbes in or on the body. An antiseptic (choice A) is a solution that kills microbes on the skin or body surface. Minerals (choice C) are a naturally occurring essential resource for the body to perform necessary functions. An asepsis (choice D) is the absence of infections or pathogens.

60. **The correct answer is B.** Using sounds to share information with others is a form of verbal communication. Cues (choice A), pictures (choice C), and facial or body movements (choice D) are all forms of non-verbal communication.

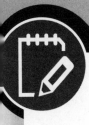

NOTES

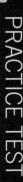

PART V

HELPFUL INFORMATION FOR PROSPECTIVE CNAs AND HHAs

| Appendix

APPENDIX

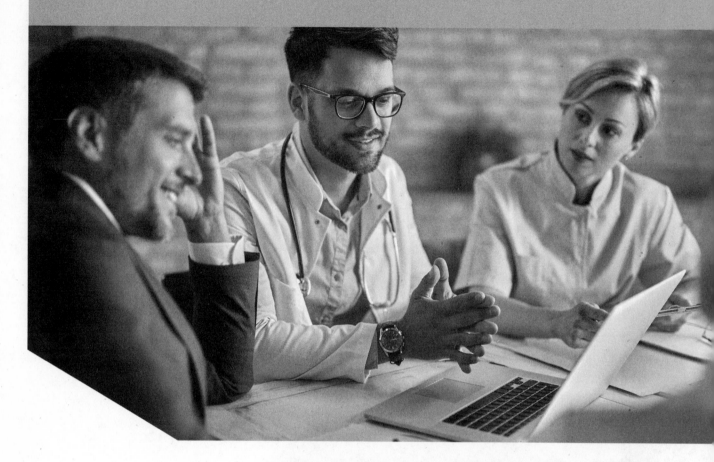

HELPFUL INFORMATION FOR PROSPECTIVE CNAs AND HHAs

The National Council of State Boards of Nursing (NCSBN) is an independent, not-for-profit organization through which nursing regulatory bodies act and counsel together on matters of common interest and concern affecting public health, safety, and welfare, including the development of nursing licensure examinations. You can access information about your state's CNA & HHA education and testing requirements on their website at **ncsbn.org.**

State Boards of Nursing

The following is a list of the state boards of nursing in the United States. If your state's education and testing requirements are mandated by your individual state rather than by a national council or test provider, contact your state's board of nursing to find out how to obtain certification as an HHA, CNA, or other nursing professional.

ALABAMA

Alabama Board of Nursing
RSA Plaza
770 Washington Avenue, Suite 250
Montgomery, AL 36104
Phone: 334-242-4060
Fax: 334-242-4360
Website: www.abn.state.al.us

ALASKA

Alaska Board of Nursing
550 West 7th Avenue, Suite 1500
Anchorage, AK 99501-3567
Phone: 907-269-8160
Fax: 907-269-8195
Website: www.commerce.alaska.gov/web/cbpl/
ProfessionalLicensing/BoardofNursing.aspx

ARIZONA

Arizona State Board of Nursing
1740 W Adams Street, Suite 2000
Phoenix, AZ 85007
Phone: 602-771-7800
Website: www.azbn.gov

ARKANSAS

Arkansas State Board of Nursing
University Tower Building
1123 South University Avenue, Suite 800
Little Rock, AR 72204-1619
Phone: 501-686-2700
Fax: 501-686-2714
Website: https://www.healthy.arkansas.gov/programs-
services/topics/arkansas-board-of-nursing

CALIFORNIA

California State Board of Registered Nursing
1747 N. Market Blvd., Suite 150
Sacramento, CA 95834-1924
Phone: 916-322-3350
Fax: 916-574-7699
Website: www.rn.ca.gov

COLORADO

Colorado Board of Nursing
1560 Broadway, Suite 1350
Denver, CO 80202
Phone: 303-894-2430
Fax: 303-894-2821
Website: dpo.colorado.gov/Nursing

CONNECTICUT

Connecticut Board of Examiners for Nursing
Department of Public Health
410 Capitol Avenue, MS#13PHO
Hartford, CT 06134-0328
Phone: 860-509-7603
Fax: 860-509-8457
Website: https://portal.ct.gov/DPH/Public-Health-Hearing-
Office/Board-of-Examiners-for-Nursing/Board-of-
Examiners-for-Nursing

DELAWARE

Delaware Board of Nursing
Cannon Building
861 Silver Lake Blvd., Suite 203
Dover, DE 19904
Phone: 302-739-4500
Fax: 302-739-2711
Website: http://dpr.delaware.gov/boards/nursing

DISTRICT OF COLUMBIA

District of Columbia Board of Nursing
Department of Health
Health Professional Licensing Administration
899 North Capitol Street, NE
Washington, DC 20002
Phone: 202-442-5955
Fax: 202-442-4795
Website: https://dchealth.dc.gov/bon

FLORIDA

Florida Board of Nursing
4052 Bald Cypress Way, Bin C-02
Tallahassee, FL 32399-3252
Phone: 850-245-4125
Website: www.floridanursing.gov

GEORGIA

Georgia Board of Nursing
237 Coliseum Drive
Macon, GA 31217-3858
Phone: 844-753-7825
Fax: 877-371-5712
Website: https://sos.ga.gov/index.php/licensing/plb/45

HAWAII

Hawaii Board of Nursing
Professional and Vocational Licensing Division
Attn: Board of Nursing
P.O. Box 3469
Honolulu, HI 96801
Phone: 808-586-3000
Fax: 808-586-2689
Website: http://hawaii.gov/dcca/areas/pvi/boards/nursing

IDAHO

Idaho Board of Nursing
280 North 8th Street, Suite 210
Boise, ID 83720-0061
Phone: 208-334-3110
Fax: 208-334-3262
Website: https://ibn.idaho.gov/

ILLINOIS

Illinois Board of Nursing
James R. Thompson Center
100 West Randolph, Suite 9-300
Chicago, IL 60601
Phone: 312-814-2715
Fax: 312-814-3145
Website: www.idfpr.com/profs/Nursing.asp

INDIANA

Indiana Professional Licensing Agency
Attn: Indiana State Board of Nursing
402 West Washington Street, Room W072
Indianapolis, IN 46204
Phone: 317-234-2043
Fax: 317-233-4236
Website: www.in.gov/pla/nursing.htm

IOWA

Iowa Board of Nursing
400 S.W. 8th Street, Suite B
Des Moines, IA 50309-4685
Phone: 515-281-3255
Fax: 515-281-4825
Website: https://nursing.iowa.gov

KANSAS

Kansas State Board of Nursing
Landon State Office Building
900 SW Jackson Street, Suite 1051
Topeka, KS 66612-1230
Phone: 785-296-4929
Fax: 785-296-3929
Website: www.ksbn.org

KENTUCKY

Kentucky Board of Nursing
312 Whittington Parkway, Suite 300
Louisville, KY 40222
Phone: 502-429-3300
Fax: 502-429-3311
Website: http://kbn.ky.gov

LOUISIANA

Louisiana State Board of Nursing
17373 Perkins Road
Baton Rouge, LA 70810
Phone: 225-755-7500
Fax: 225-755-7584
Website: www.lsbn.state.la.us

MAINE

Maine State Board of Nursing
161 Capitol Street
158 State House Station
Augusta, ME 04333-0158
Phone: 207-287-1133
Fax: 207-287-1149
Website: www.maine.gov/boardofnursing

MARYLAND

Maryland Board of Nursing
4140 Patterson Avenue
Baltimore, MD 21215-2254
Phone: 410-585-1900
Fax: 410-358-3530
Website: https://mbon.maryland.gov/Pages/default.aspx

MASSACHUSETTS

Massachusetts State Nursing Board
Commonwealth of Massachusetts
239 Causeway Street, Suite 500
Boston, MA 02114
Phone: 800-414-0168
Fax: 617-973-0984
Website: http://mass.gov/dph/boards/rn

MICHIGAN

Office of Health Services
Michigan Department of Licensing and Regulatory Affairs
611 W. Ottawa
P.O. Box 30004
Lansing, MI 48909
Phone: 517-373-9102
Fax: 517-373-2179
Website: www.michigan.gov/lara

MINNESOTA

Minnesota Board of Nursing
2829 University Avenue SE, Suite 500
Minneapolis, MN 55414
Phone: 612-317-3000
Fax: 612-617-2190
Website: www.nursingboard.state.mn.us

MISSISSIPPI

Mississippi Board of Nursing
713 Pear Orchard Road, Plaza II, Suite 300
Ridgeland, MS 39157
Phone: 601-957-6300
Fax: 601-957-6301
Website: www.msbn.state.ms.us

MISSOURI

Missouri State Board of Nursing
3605 Missouri Boulevard
P.O. Box 656
Jefferson City, MO 65102-0656
Phone: 573-751-0681
Fax: 573-751-0075
Website: http://pr.mo.gov/nursing.asp

MONTANA

Montana State Board of Nursing
P.O. Box 200513
Helena, MT 59620-0513
Phone: 406-444-6880
Website: http://boards.bsd.dli.mt.gov/nur

NEBRASKA

Office of Nursing and Nursing Support
DHHS, Division of Public Health
Licensure Unit 301
Centennial Mall South
Lincoln, NE 68509-4986
Phone: 402-471-4376
Fax: 402-742-2360
Website: http://dhhs.ne.gov/licensure/Pages/Nurse-Licensing.aspx

NEVADA

Nevada State Board of Nursing
License Certification and Education
4220 S. Maryland Pkwy., Building B, Suite 300
Las Vegas, NV 89119-7533
Phone: 702-486-5803
Website: https://nevadanursingboard.org

NEW HAMPSHIRE

New Hampshire Board of Nursing
121 South Fruit Street, Suite 102
Concord, NH 03301
Phone: 603-271-2323
Fax: 603-271-6605
Website: www.oplc.nh.gov/nursing

NEW JERSEY

New Jersey Board of Nursing
124 Halsey Street, 6th Floor
Newark, NJ 07102
Phone: 973-504-6430
Website: www.njconsumeraffairs.gov/nur/Pages/default.
aspx

NEW MEXICO

New Mexico Board of Nursing
6301 Indian School Road NE, Suite 710
Albuquerque, NM 87110
Phone: 505-841-8340
Fax: 505-841-8347
Website: http://nmbon.sks.com

NEW YORK

New York State Board of Nursing
Education Building
89 Washington Avenue
2nd Floor West Wing
Albany, NY 12234
Phone: 518-474-3817, Ext. 120
Fax: 518-474-3706
Website: https://www.ncsbn.org/New%20York.htm

NORTH CAROLINA

North Carolina Board of Nursing
3724 National Drive, Suite 201
Raleigh, NC 27612
Phone: 919-782-3211
Fax: 919-781-9461
Website: www.ncbon.com

NORTH DAKOTA

North Dakota Board of Nursing
919 South 7th Street, Suite 504
Bismarck, ND 58504
Phone: 701-328-9777
Fax: 701-328-9785
Website: www.ndbon.org

OHIO

Ohio Board of Nursing
17 South High Street, Suite 660
Columbus, OH 43215-3466
Phone: 614-466-3947
Fax: 614-466-0388
Website: www.nursing.ohio.gov

OKLAHOMA

Oklahoma Board of Nursing
2915 North Classen Boulevard, Suite 524
Oklahoma City, OK 73106
Phone: 405-962-1800
Fax: 405-962-1821
Website: www.nursing.ok.gov

OREGON

Oregon State Board of Nursing
17938 SW Upper Boones Ferry Rd.
Portland, OR 97224
Phone: 971-673-0685
Website: https://www.oregon.gov/osbn/Pages/index.aspx

PENNSYLVANIA

Pennsylvania State Board of Nursing
Penn Center
2601 N 3rd Street
Harrisburg, PA 17110
Phone: 717-787-8503
Fax: 717-783-0510
Website: www.dos.state.pa.us/bpoa/site/default.asp

RHODE ISLAND

Rhode Island Board of Nurse
Registration and Nursing Education
105 Cannon Building, Three Capitol Hill
Providence, RI 02908
Phone: 401-222-5700
Fax: 401-222-3352
Website: www.health.ri.gov/licenses/detail.php?id=231

SOUTH CAROLINA

South Carolina State Board of Nursing
Synergy Business Park
Kingstree Building
110 Centerview Drive
Columbia, SC 29210
Phone: 803-896-4300
Website: https://llr.sc.gov/nurse/

SOUTH DAKOTA

South Dakota Board of Nursing
4305 South Louise Avenue, Suite 201
Sioux Falls, SD 57106-3305
Phone: 605-362-2760
Fax: 605-362-2768
Website: http://doh.sd.gov/boards/nursing

TENNESSEE

Tennessee Board of Nursing
665 Mainstream Drive, 2nd Floor
Nashville, TN 37243
Phone: 1-800-778-4123
Website: www.tn.gov/health/health-program-areas/
health-professional-boards/nursing-board/nursing-board/
about.html

TEXAS

Texas Board of Nurse Examiners
333 Guadalupe, Suite 3-460
Austin, TX 78701-3944
Phone: 512-305-7400
Fax: 512-305-7401
Website: www.bne.state.tx.us

UTAH

Utah State Board of Nursing
Heber M. Wells Building, 4th Floor
160 East 300 South
Salt Lake City, UT 84111
Phone: 801-530-6628
Fax: 801-530-6511
Website: https://dopl.utah.gov/nurse/index.html

VERMONT

Office of Professional Regulation
Board of Nursing
89 Main Street, Floor 3
Montpelier, VT 05620-3402
Phone: 802-828-2396
Fax: 802-828-2484
Website: https://sos.vermont.gov/nursing/

VIRGINIA

Virginia Board of Nursing
Dept of Health Professions
Perimeter Center
9960 Mayland Drive, Suite 300
Richmond, VA 23233-1463
Phone: 804-367-4515
Fax: 804-527-4455
Website: www.dhp.virginia.gov/Boards/Nursing/

WASHINGTON

Washington State Nursing Care
Quality Assurance Commission
111 Israel Rd SE
Tumwater, WA 98501
Phone: 360-236-4703
Fax: 360-236-4738
Website: www.doh.wa.gov/LicensesPermitsandCertificates/
NursingCommission

WEST VIRGINIA

West Virginia Board of Examiners for Registered
Professional Nurses
90 MacCorkle Ave. SW, Suite 203
South Charleston, WV 25303
Phone: 304-744-0900
Fax: 304-744-0600
Website: www.wvrnboard.com

WISCONSIN

Wisconsin Department of Regulation and Licensing
4822 Madison Yards Way
Madison, WI 53705
Phone: 608-266-2112
Fax: 608-266-2264
Website: https://dsps.wi.gov/Pages/Professions/RN/Default.
aspx

WYOMING

Wyoming State Board of Nursing
130 Hobbs Ave, Ste B
Cheyenne, WY 82002
Phone: 307-777-7601
Fax: 307-777-3519
Website: http://nursing.state.wy.us

notes

notes

notes

notes

notes

notes

notes

notes

notes

notes

notes

notes

notes

notes

notes

notes

notes